THE
RADIOLOGY
HANDBOOK

A Pocket Guide to Medical Imaging

J. S. Benseler, D.O.

A WHITE COAT POCKET GUIDE
Series editor John A. Brose, D.O.

Ohio University Press

in association with the
Ohio University College of
Osteopathic Medicine

ATHENS

T0132976

Ohio University Press, Athens, Ohio 45701
www.ohio.edu/oupress
© 2006 by Ohio University Press

Ohio University Press books are printed on acid-free paper ® ™

13 12 11 10 09   5 4 3

Library of Congress Cataloging-in-Publication Data

Benseler, J. S., 1954-
The radiology handbook : a pocket guide to medical imaging / J.S. Benseler.
    p. ; cm. — (White coat pocket guide series)
Includes bibliographical references and index.
ISBN-13: 978-0-8214-1708-9 (pbk : alk. paper)
ISBN-10: 0-8214-1708-8 (pbk : alk. paper)
 1. Radiology, Medical—Handbooks, manuals, etc. 2. Diagnosis, Radioscopic—Handbooks, manuals, etc.
3. Imaging systems in medicine—Handbooks, manuals, etc. I. Title. II. Series: White coat pocket guide.
    [DNLM: 1. Diagnostic Imaging—methods—Handbooks. WN 39 B47r 2006]
RM847.B46 2006
616.07'57—dc22
                                                              2006015339

Contents

Preface

The Radiology Handbook provides a foundation for the study of radiology. It is designed to serve as a basic introduction to medical image interpretation for medical students and nonradiologists. This pocket reference is organized into three parts: ordering schemes, general information, and practice images.

You should use the ordering scheme in part 1 of this book as a general guide for requesting the appropriate test for a given clinical presentation. This section is organized anatomically from head to toe.

If you are just beginning to study (or restudy) radiology, you should start by learning the basics of how an image is formed. The first four chapters in part 2 provide the foundation for understanding how images are created by X-rays, CT, ultrasound, and MRI. Chapters 5 through 11 contain basic information pertaining to ordering and interpretation in the chest, abdomen, urinary tract, GI system, musculoskeletal system, head and neck, and nervous system. All chapters are arranged in a question-and-answer format. Chapter 12 is a brief discussion of how to become more comfortable and proficient with image interpretation. Part 3 provides an opportunity for self-testing. Images of normal anatomy and common imaging pathology are followed by an answer key.

The Radiology Handbook is not intended to be comprehensive. I like to refer to the information provided in this guide as a "punch in the nose." It's not the whole fight, but it's a good beginning. The information is purposefully succinct—a quick read for busy physicians-in-training. I wish you all the best as you evolve into excellent diagnosticians.

PART ONE

Ordering Schemes

The following is a list of patient symptoms accompanied by the imaging studies that may be beneficial for arriving at an accurate diagnosis. Please understand that there may never be universal consensus among clinicians about the imaging study that is best in any given clinical circumstance. The following recommendations are based on my own clinical experience as well as guidelines from current literature. When in doubt, always consult with the radiologist.

Ordering Schemes

BODY AREA	**SYMPTOM/CONDITION**	**IMAGING STUDIES**
Brain	Aneurysm	MRI/MRA Catheter cerebral angiography
	Difficulty speaking	Noncontrast head CT and/or Cranial MRI with diffusion imaging
	Double vision	Pre- and postcontrast MRI (attention orbits, optic nerves, tracts, and optic radiations)
	Fever/headache	Pre- and postcontrast CT and/or Pre- and postcontrast MRI
	Hearing loss	CT of temporal bones and/or Cranial MRI attention IACs
	Hemorrhagic stroke	Noncontrast head CT followed by MRI
	Ischemic stroke	Noncontrast head CT (may miss stroke in first 24 hours) MRI with diffusion imaging Perfusion imaging (MRI)
	Mastoid infection/tumor	CT of temporal bones

Memory loss	Pre- and postcontrast CT and/or Cranial MRI
Middle-ear infection	CT of temporal bones
Multiple sclerosis	Pre- and postcontrast MRI
Ringing in the ears	Pre- and postcontrast MRI (attention internal auditory canals)
Seizure	Cranial MRI (attention medial temporal lobes) and PET
Severe headache	Pre- and postcontrast CT or Pre- and postcontrast MRI
Stiff neck	Noncontrast head CT Pre- and postcontrast MRI
Trauma	Noncontrast head CT
Vascular malformation	MRA and/or Catheter cerebral angiography
Visual field defect	Pre- and postcontrast MRI (attention orbits, optic nerves, tracts, and optic radiations)

Ordering Schemes

BODY AREA	SYMPTOM/CONDITION	IMAGING STUDIES
Brain *(cont.)*	Weakness/paralysis	Head CT and/or Cranial MRI with diffusion imaging
Head	Acute sinusitis	No imaging indicated Exceptions: suspect brain abscess, tumor, nonresponse to therapy
	Facial bone trauma	X-ray and/or noncontrast facial bone CT
	Nasal bone trauma	X-ray
	Orbital trauma	X-ray and/or Noncontrast orbit CT
	Skull fracture	Head CT with bone window settings Skull X-ray
	Unresolving sinusitis	Sinus CT

Neck	Enlarged thyroid	Nuclear thyroid uptake/scan and Ultrasound
	Epiglottitis	AP and lateral neck X-ray
	Lymphadenopathy	CT or MRI
	Mass unknown etiology	CT (without/with contrast) or MRI
	Retropharyngeal abscess	CT
	Salivary gland mass	CT or MRI
	Sialolithiasis	CT (without/with contrast)
	Stridor	AP and lateral neck X-ray
	Thyroid nodule	Nuclear thyroid uptake/scan and Ultrasound
	Vocal nodule	CT

Ordering Schemes

BODY AREA	SYMPTOM/CONDITION	IMAGING STUDIES
Chest	Aortic aneurysm	Chest CT/CTA/angiography
	Aortic dissection	Aortic MRI or chest CT and/or angiography Transesophageal echography
	Chest pain	Chest X-ray Expiratory PA if suspect pneumothorax CTA if suspect PE
	Cough/fever	Chest X-ray
	Dyspnea	Chest X-ray
	Esophageal rupture	Chest CT
	Hemoptysis	Chest CT
	Lung nodule/mass	Chest CT followed by PET
	Occupational exposure	Chest X-ray Chest CT (high resolution)
	Orthopnea	Chest X-ray

	Pleural effusion	Chest X-ray with decubitus
		Ultrasound (guided thoracentesis)
		Chest CT (malignant effusion)
	Trauma	Chest X-ray/Chest CT
	Unresolving cough	Chest CT
	Wheezing	Chest X-ray
		Expiratory if suspect foreign body

Esophagus	Cancer	Esophagram and CT thorax
	Diverticulum	Esophagram
	Dysphagia	Esophagram/CT
	Foreign body	Esophagram
	Reflux/heartburn	Esophagram

Ordering Schemes

BODY AREA	SYMPTOM/CONDITION	IMAGING STUDIES
Abdomen	Adrenal pathology	Abdomen CT with contrast
	Ascites	Abdomen CT or Abdominal ultrasound
	Bleeding, GI	Nuclear RBC study (0.1 cc/min rate of blood loss) Angiography (1.0 cc/min blood loss)
	Cholecystitis	Ultrasound/HIDA scan
	Cirrhosis	Hepatic CT Ultrasound for ascites Esophagram for varices
	Colon obstruction	Abdominal X-ray Barium enema (water soluble)
	Crohn's disease	CT, MRI, or small bowel follow-through
	Epigastric pain	Abdomen CT or abdomen ultrasound
	Flank pain	Noncontrast renal CT Renal ultrasound Intravenous pyelogram

Gallstone	Ultrasound
Hemangioma (liver)	Hepatic CT (hemangioma protocol) Nuclear SPECT imaging MRI
Intussusception	Air-only enema (children) Barium enema (adults)
Jaundice	Abdomen CT or Abdominal ultrasound and/or Nuclear HIDA scan Magnetic resonance cholangiogram ERCP
Meckel's diverticulitis	Abdomen-pelvis CT Pertechnetate scintigraphy Tc-99m
Pain (nonspecific)	Acute abdominal series Abdomen CT if persistent
RLQ pain (appendicitis)	Ultrasound (children) Abdomen CT (adults)

Ordering Schemes

BODY AREA	SYMPTOM/CONDITION	IMAGING STUDIES
Abdomen *(cont.)*	RUQ pain	GB ultrasound
	Small bowel obstruction	Abdomen X-ray Small bowel follow-through
	Splenic trauma	Abdomen CT
	Trauma	Abdomen CT Ultrasound (if patient is unstable)
Pelvis	Dysmenorrhea	Pelvic ultrasound
	Hip pain (AVN)	X-ray followed by hip MRI
	LLQ pain (diverticulitis)	Abdomen-pelvis CT
	Pelvic pain	Pelvic ultrasound Pelvic CT or MRI
	Prostate cancer staging	Pelvic MRI
	Trauma	X-ray and CT

	Uterine cancer staging	Pelvic MRI
Scrotum	Pain/swelling/mass	Scrotal ultrasound
	Testicular torsion	Scrotal ultrasound with Doppler
Perineum	Pain/trauma/infection	Pelvic CT

Shoulder	A-C separation	X-ray (option: weight holding)
	Brachial plexopathy	MRI
	Clavicle fracture	X-ray
	Dislocation	Shoulder X-ray
	Glenoid labrum tear	MRI arthrography
	Glenoid/scapular fracture	CT with 3D reconstruction
	Persistent pain	MRI (option MR arthrography)

Ordering Schemes

BODY AREA	**SYMPTOM/CONDITION**	**IMAGING STUDIES**
Shoulder *(cont.)*	Recurrent dislocation	MRI
	Rotator cuff tear	MRI
	Trauma	X-ray CT for fracture MRI for soft tissue injury
Upper arm	Mass (soft tissue or bone)	MRI
	Trauma or foreign body	X-ray
Elbow	Mass or infection	MRI, bone scan (three phase)
	Tendon/ligament tear	MRI
	Trauma or foreign body	X-ray CT for complex fractures
Forearm	Mass or infection	MRI
	Trauma or foreign body	X-ray

Wrist	Carpal tunnel syndrome	MRI
	Ligament disruption	MRI
	Soft tissue injury, Mass or Infection	MRI
	Trauma or foreign body	X-ray CT Nuclear imaging for occult fracture
Hand	Infection	MRI Three-phase nuclear bone scan Nuclear white blood cell scan
	Soft tissue injury, Mass	MRI
	Trauma or foreign body	X-ray

Ordering Schemes

BODY AREA	SYMPTOM/CONDITION	IMAGING STUDIES
Hip	Acetabulum fracture	X-ray, CT with 3D reconstruction
	Infection	MRI Three-phase nuclear bone scan Nuclear white blood cell scan
	Legg-Perthes	MRI
	Pain (AVN)	MRI
	Trauma	X-ray, MRI, nuclear bone scan, CT
Femur	Infection	Three-phase nuclear bone scan or white cell study (nuclear)
	Mass	MRI
	Trauma	X-ray
Knee	Baker's cyst	Ultrasound or MRI
	Infection	MRI Three-phase nuclear bone scan Nuclear white blood cell scan

	Ligament/meniscus tear	MRI
	Swelling/effusion	MRI
	Trauma	X-ray CT for tibial plateau fracture
	Tumor	X-ray and MRI
Lower leg	Infection	MRI Three-phase nuclear bone scan Nuclear white blood cell scan
	Mass	MRI
	Trauma/foreign body	X-ray
Ankle	Avascular necrosis	MRI
	Infection	MRI Three-phase nuclear bone scan Nuclear white blood cell scan

Ordering Schemes

BODY AREA	SYMPTOM/CONDITION	IMAGING STUDIES
Ankle *(cont.)*	Ligament injury	MRI
	Mass	MRI
	Tendonopathy	MRI
	Trauma	X-ray CT if complex fracture
Foot	Infection	MRI Three-phase nuclear bone scan Nuclear white blood cell scan
	Ligament injury	MRI
	Mass	MRI
	Morton's neuroma	MRI
	Plantar fasciitis	MRI
	Tarsal coalition	CT with 3D reconstruction
	Trauma	X-ray CT if calcaneus fracture

Toe	Infection	MRI
		Three-phase nuclear bone scan
		Nuclear white blood cell scan
	Mass	MRI
	Trauma	X-ray
Vascular	Aneurysm or AVM	CTA, MRA, and/or angiography
	Deep vein thrombosis	Doppler ultrasound
		Magnetic resonance venography
	Hypertension	Renal scan and flow study and
		Renal CTA or Renal MRA
	Peripheral vascular disease	CTA, MRA, and/or angiography (claudication)

Ordering Schemes

CT/MRI Comparison

	MRI BEST	MRI = CT	CT BEST
Head and neck	Vascular lesions	Hydrocephalus	Acute hemorrhage
	Seizures	Headache screening	Head trauma
	Acoustic neuroma	Cerebral infarction	Orbits
	Primary neoplasia	Parathyroid	Paranasal sinuses
	Metastasis	Nasopharynx	Calcified lesions
	Infections	Salivary glands	Middle ear
	Pituitary lesions		Acute headache
	Multiple sclerosis		Larynx
	Neuro-degenerative		
	Venous thrombosis		
	Dementia		
	Congenital anomaly		
Thorax	Cardiac masses	Aortic dissection	Hilar mass
		Pericardium	Lung nodule
		Mediastinum	COPD
			Pulmonary fibrosis
			Asbestosis

			Pneumoconiosis
			Persistent pneumonia
			Pulmonary embolism
			Pleural effusion
			Mesothelioma
Abdomen	Hemangioma	Liver metastasis	Liver
	Venous thrombosis	Renal tumors	Spleen
	Hemochromatosis	Aortic disease	Pancreas
		Hemangioma	Kidney
			Adrenal
			Trauma
			Lymphadenopathy
			Abscess
Pelvis	Uterine fibroid	Cervical cancer*	Adenopathy
	Endometrium*	Rectal cancer*	Diverticulitis
	Prostate cancer*	Ovarian cancer*	Appendicitis
		Bladder cancer*	

*Cancer staging.

Ordering Schemes

	MRI BEST	**MRI = CT**	**CT BEST**
Musculo- Skeletal	Hip AVN		Joint fracture
	Marrow disorders		Joint loose body
	Shoulder		
	Knee		
	Bone neoplasm		
	Soft tissue neoplasm		
	TMJ		
	Osteomyelitis		
	Ankle		
	Elbow		
	Wrist/hand		
	Ligaments		
	Cartilage		
Spine	Congenital anomaly	Lumbar radiculopathy	Spondylosis
	Radiculopathy	Spinal stenosis	Bone abnormality
	Myelopathy	Vertebral fracture	Spinal trauma
	Neoplasia		
	Syrinx		
	Spinal cord		
	Scar vs. HNP		
	Infection		

PART TWO

Imaging Overview

CHAPTER ONE   X-RAYS

1.0 Goals: Understanding and working with X-rays

Objective questions:

1.1   What is an X-ray?
1.2   How can X-rays produce images of internal structures of the body?
1.3   What are the five basic radiographic densities?
1.4   What are the three key elements of radiation safety?
1.5   What is a safe dose of radiation?
1.6   What can happen when people are exposed to radiation?
1.7   Are there special considerations for children?
1.8   How do I order an X-ray?
1.9   How do I develop a differential diagnosis?
1.10 Is there an optimal way to view a radiograph?
1.11 What is the basic analysis of any structure or mass?

1.1 What Is an X-ray?

X-rays are a form of electromagnetic energy formed when high-speed electrons bombard a tungsten anode target. Like light energy, these useful rays have properties of waves and particles. However, X-rays have a much shorter wavelength than visible light, allowing them to penetrate matter.

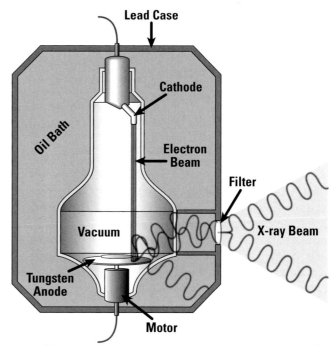

X-ray machine

X-rays

1.2 How can X-rays produce images of internal structures of the body?

Differences in body tissue densities are what allow us to "see" inside the body by creating a shadowgram. The body is composed of tissues containing many different elements, which vary by atomic number (the number of protons in the nucleus). The higher the atomic number, the denser the element and the more effectively the X-ray is blocked. Therefore, specific shadows of internal body structures become visible because they contain varying types of elements. For example, when an X-ray strikes the calcium in cortical bone, it is blocked, and on the radiographic image the bone will appear white. When an X-ray strikes a less dense element like nitrogen, it passes all the way through. Therefore, the air-containing lungs will appear darker, approaching black on the radiographic image. When a fracture extends through bone, the fracture line will be dark while the intact bone will remain white.

1.3 What are the five basic radiographic densities?

Metal (Bright white)
Mineral (White)
Fluid/soft tissue (Gray)
Fat (Dark gray)
Air (Black)

> **KEY POINT**
> The higher the atomic number of the matter, the more the X-rays will be blocked from reaching the film. (N = atomic number = number of protons in the atom of an element.)

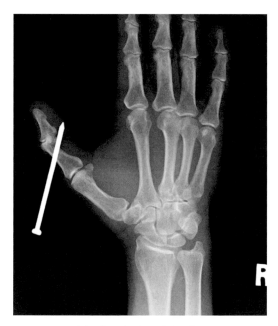

Metal and mineral density

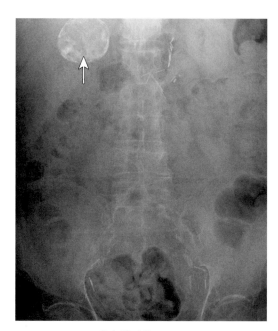

Calcified liver cyst

X-rays

1.4 What are the three key elements of radiation safety?

The first element of radiation safety is *time*. As health care providers, we must limit the amount of time that we and our patients are exposed to radiation. The second element of safety is *distance*. The energy and therefore potential damage caused by X-rays are inversely proportional to the distance squared. The farther we are from the source of radiation, the safer we are. The third element of safety is *shielding*. By covering the body with a protective metallic shield, we can effectively limit the dose of radiation to that part of the body.

> *The three elements of radiation safety*
>
> *Time* (Reduce to a minimum the time you spend around an X-ray source)
> *Distance* (X-ray dose is inversely proportional to the distance squared)
> *Shielding* (Aprons composed of metal that block X-rays)

1.5 What is a safe dose of radiation?

There is no dose of radiation that is considered perfectly safe. We are all exposed to ambient radiation in the environment. It comes from the sun and other celestial bodies and from the ground, including a well-known source—radon. Unnecessary exposure from imaging studies is a preventable hazard. Always consider risk versus benefit when requesting any test utilizing radiation.

1.6 What can happen when people are exposed to radiation?

X-rays can dislodge electrons from the shell of an atom. This results in the production of an ion (free radical). A free radical is an unstable molecule with an extra electron. Free radicals become stable by donating their extra electron to other molecules within cells of the body. This process permanently damages protein, DNA and other vital molecules. Among the ill effects reported from radiation exposure are birth defects, cancer and cataracts. For more information about radiation damage, dosages, and ways to protect yourself and your patients, please visit the Web site of the Nuclear Regulatory Commission, http://www.nrc.gov.

1.7 Are there special considerations for children?

Children are more vulnerable to radiation because of their rapidly dividing cells and incompletely differentiated cells. I always insist that my own children be well covered by a protective apron whenever they have an X-ray study. To be sure that your pediatric, adolescent, and young adult patients are shielded, always indicate on the order that shielding is requested. Technologists are taught to do this, but a reminder never hurts. Gonadal shielding should be used for anyone in the reproductive age group. This age range may be from 10 to 70—ask the patient! When in doubt, always shield. For medical personnel (and that includes students, interns, and residents), I recommend using a thyroid shield in addition to a protective body apron.

X-rays

1.8 How do I order an X-ray?

It is important for completeness and accuracy that physician orders follow a reproducible sequence. In the list of orders, lab and X-ray can be grouped together under the umbrella of diagnostic studies. Please note that you will be asked to provide a diagnosis when you order a study. The more information you provide, the more likely we will be to arrive at the correct imaging diagnosis.

> *Example*
>
> 1. Admit to the service of Dr. Smith
> 2. Admitting diagnosis: Pneumonia and dehydration
> 3. Activity: Bathroom privileges with assistance
> 4. Diet: Regular diet
> 5. Diagnostic studies:
>   Laboratory
>   Imaging:
>   PA and lateral chest X-ray, rule out pneumonia

1.9 Is there an optimal way to view a radiograph?

The conventional way to view any radiograph is as if you are looking at the patient from the front, in the anatomic position. Your hospital or clinic may have a picture archival and communication system (PACS). With this system, the X-ray images will appear on a computer screen. Strive to view these digital images in a dark, quiet environment. If you are viewing conventional X-ray films, always use a dedicated view box. Holding films up to an overhead light is a great way to miss something important. You and I are responsible for everything on the film, so be sure to look at all of the structures and each corner of the image.

To get the optimal ratio of light coming from the image relative to the background, a darkened room is critical. This is why movie theaters become nearly pitch-black before the movie begins. Light pollution can severely impair your ability to perceive an abnormality.

Once you have identified the shadow of a structure, whether it is a normal anatomic structure or pathology, carefully examine it for size, shape, position, and density. The questions you must ask yourself are: Is this structure normal anatomy? Is this structure abnormally large or small? Can its borders be recognized so that a measurement of size can be made? What is the shape of the structure? Where is it located, and is this a normal position? What is the radiographic density of the structure (remember the five basic radiographic densities)?

Basic concept: Analysis of any structure or mass on a radiograph

1. Size of the structure
2. Shape or contour of a structure
3. Position of the structure
4. Density of the structure

   Note: In general, a mass or nodule is more likely to be benign if it is small, smoothly marginated, and calcified. A mass or nodule is more likely to be malignant if it is large, irregular in contour, and dense but not calcified.

X-rays

1.10 How will I know if the X-ray is of diagnostic quality?

As physicians, we are responsible not only for the pathology present on an X-ray, but also for ensuring good-quality images through feedback to and supervision of the technologists who perform the studies. An overpenetrated (overexposed) radiograph is too dark. X-rays can penetrate through subtle pathology and obscure an important finding. A malignant pulmonary nodule may be difficult or impossible to see if the film is overpenetrated. An underpenetrated (underexposed) radiograph can make normal structures such as bronchovascular structures in the lungs look like pathology. The image is too light or white-looking. Sometimes a patient suspected to have congestive heart failure based on an underpenetrated radiograph may be treated for CHF unnecessarily.

The patient should be orthogonal to the X-ray beam on a PA or AP view. This means that the beam enters the patient at 90 degrees and there is no patient rotation. On a well-positioned PA chest X-ray, the spinous process at T1 should be equidistant from the medial ends of the clavicles.

Watch out for artifacts. Objects in clothing and hair and on the skin create shadows that can mimic pathology. A patient who was sent for a chest X-ray was chewing a piece of gum, which he put on his upper back for safe keeping. The resulting nodular-appearing opacity caused quite a stir until the patient was examined and the cause of the "lesion" was revealed.

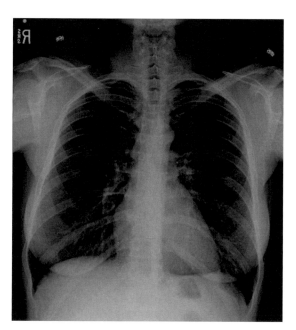

Overpenetrated chest X-ray

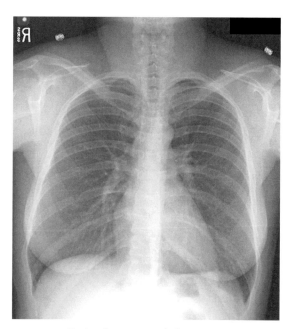

Optimally penetrated chest X-ray

X-rays

1.11 How can I develop a differential diagnosis?

Occasionally (not often enough, as far as I'm concerned) a diagnosis is obvious. The late Dr. Felson, a brilliant mind in radiology, called these recognizable X-ray findings "Aunt Minnie." Aunt Minnie is the relative whom we may see once every 10 years, but whose appearance is so characteristic that we know her the minute we see her. There is an excellent Web site for radiology education called http://AuntMinnie.com. Examples of Aunt Minnie include such entities as calcification of the gallbladder wall in the condition known as porcelain gallbladder, or laminated calcified gallstones or a staghorn renal calculus. Most of the time we must create a list of possible diagnoses. Radiographic findings are not specific. To arrive at the correct diagnosis, history, physical, laboratory, and imaging data must be correlated.

For guiding students through the general disease categories to be considered in a differential diagnosis, I like the mnemonic "VITAMINS D and C":

V = Vascular
I = Infection or Inflammation
T = Trauma
A = Autoimmune or Allergic
M = Metabolic
I = Idiopathic or Iatrogenic
N = Neoplastic
S = Structural
D = Developmental
C = Cardiac

Picture this. Your attending physician catches you off guard and asks for the differential diagnosis for a patient with an unusual pain pattern and symptom complex. Your answer may go like this:

> I've been thinking about that, Dr. Smith. I believe we have to consider the possibility of a *vascular* cause. Of course, an *infection* such as TB, the "great masquerader," should be considered, but bacterial, fungal, and viral etiologies are contained in my differential thinking. Has this patient experienced *trauma?* I always think of *autoimmune* processes in cases such as these. The endocrine system can produce a variety of *metabolic* disorders that must be considered. Have we thought about the possibility of an *iatrogenic* drug reaction? Primary and metastatic *neoplasm* can present with similar symptoms. I learned that *structure* and function are inseparably related. I would also consider a congenital or *developmental* cause in this case. If all else fails, let's make sure there is not a *cardiac* origin.

X-rays

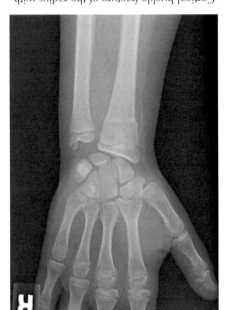

Cortical buckle fracture of the radius with ulnar styloid avulsion

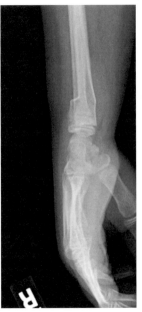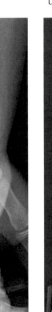

Lateral view

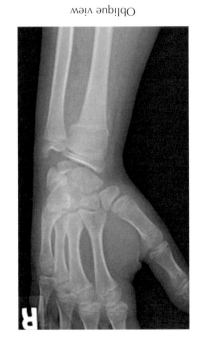

Oblique view

34

2.0 Goals: Understanding how CT works: its uses, strengths, and weaknesses

Objective questions:

2.1   What is CT?
2.2   How does CT work?
2.3   What are Hounsfield units?
2.4   Are there limitations to CT?
2.5   What are window settings and how are they used?
2.6   What parts of the body are best studied with CT?
2.7   What is contrast CT?
2.8   What are 3D CT and sagittal and coronal reconstruction?
2.9   What is CTA?
2.10 What are the benefits of CT compared to plain radiography?
2.11 What are the benefits of CT compared to MRI?

Computed Tomography

2.1 What is CT?

Computed tomography (CT) provides us with images (tomograms) showing slices through the body. We can vary the thickness of these slices so that, in effect, we are looking at thin two-dimensional pictures representing a volume of tissue. *Computed axial tomography* (CAT) is a synonym for CT. It refers to the axial plane, the most common plane of CT imaging.

2.2 How does CT work?

CT uses X-rays to produce an image. The same basic principles apply to CT as to all other X-ray studies. X-rays are blocked (attenuated) by tissues depending upon their density (atomic number). Air is black on CT and minerals are white.

To obtain a slice, an X-ray source rotates around the body in an arc while an X-ray detection source rotates opposite the source on the opposite side of the body. The computer analyzes the number and density of the transmitted X-rays, calculates the coordinates, and assigns a gray scale to individual picture elements (pixels) that will make the final picture.

2.3 What are Hounsfield units?

Sir Godfrey Hounsfield was instrumental in the development of computed tomography. His name is used for the numbers associated with the gray scale produced during CT scanning. All CT scanners are programmed such that water appears dark on the image; its attenuation value in Hounsfield units (HU) is 0. From this central point, HU range from calcium at approximately +1,000 HU to air at approximately –1,000 HU.

Common CT-assigned attenuation values:

Air = –1,000 HU or less (black)
Fat = –5 to –50 HU (dark gray)
Water = 0 HU (gray)

Soft tissue = +40 to +80 HU (light gray)
Calcium (stone) = +100 to +400 HU (gray white)
Cortical bone = +1,000 HU (white)

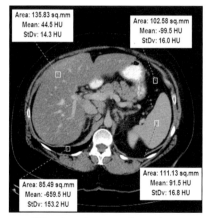

CT-assigned attenuation values

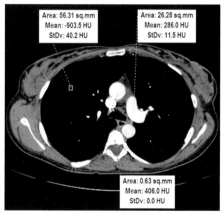

CT-assigned attenuation values:
Lung = –903.5 HU   *Contrast* = 286.0 HU
Bone = 406.0 HU

Computed Tomography

2.4 Are there limitations to CT?

CT cannot distinguish soft tissue structures as well as MRI can. For example, the ligaments and menisci of the knee are not different enough in their attenuation values to allow us to delineate them easily or demonstrate specific pathology.

Metal can create a "starburst artifact" that blurs the image. This can happen around the maxillary area and mandible due to dental fillings, as well as around the hip when a prosthesis is present.

CT is limited in the posterior fossa of the brain because of the dense bone in the petrous ridges and the skull base. A "beam-hardening artifact" limits our ability to detect subtle pathology in the brain stem area.

In addition, CT is less sensitive than MRI in the detection of white matter disease of the brain.

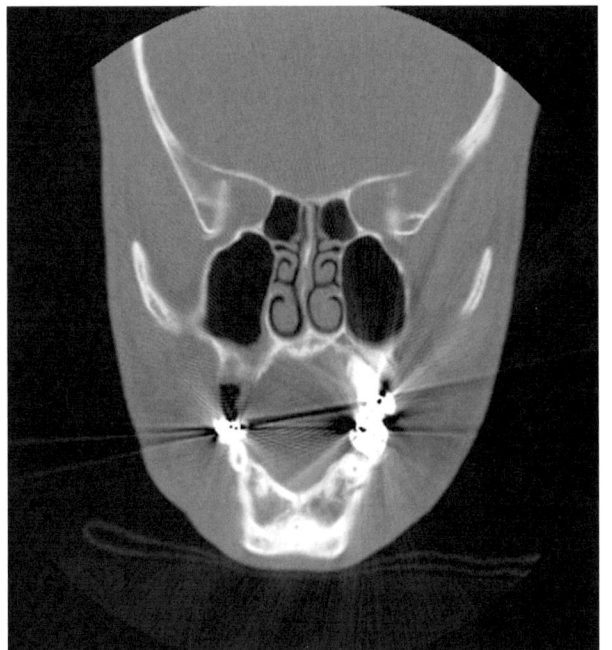

Metal artifact

2.5 What are window settings and how are they used?

Digital technology such as CT, MRI, and digital radiography provides the opportunity for computer-aided manipulation of the image. *Window widths* and *window levels* are used to optimize visualization of specific structures. The window level is the midpoint of the gray scale. The window width is the number of gray shades. If the window level is set to 0 and the window width is set to 1,000, the gray scale is from –500 to +500.

The most obvious example of windowing and leveling technique is chest CT. To evaluate the mediastinum, the window level is set to soft tissue density and the window width is set moderately narrow to allow for optimal contrast. To evaluate the lungs, the window level is set closer to air density and the window width is set relatively wide to allow detailed assessment of the air-bearing lung parenchyma.

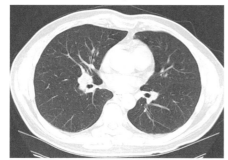

CT lung window setting

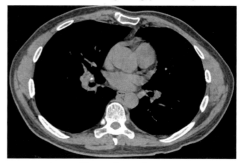

CT mediastinal window setting

Computed Tomography

2.6 What parts of the body are best studied with CT?

CT can be used from head to toe.

Head: An excellent screening modality for cranial trauma, suspected intracranial bleeding, or stroke

Paranasal sinuses

Neck

Facial bones

Chest

Abdomen

Pelvis

Knee: for evaluation of tibial plateau fractures; not good for cartilage or ligament injury evaluation

Hip: specifically for assessment of acetabulum fracture

Calcaneus: fracture

2.7 What is contrast CT?

In contrast CT, a fluid containing iodine (mineral density) is injected intravenously. Contrast is routinely employed during chest, abdomen, and pelvis CT. It helps to identify vascular structures so that they may be differentiated from other normal or abnormal structures. Contrast also helps to characterize certain types of pathology, such as infection or vascular malformations. It is not necessary to specify on the order whether you would like contrast to be administered. The exception is head CT, for which you do need to specify contrast. Contrast is indicated if you suspect primary or metastatic cancer, infection (abscess), vascular malformation, or aneurysm.

2.8 What are 3D CT and sagittal and coronal reconstruction?

Software provided on CT scanners allows for the conversion of axial images into images in any other plane desired. Three-dimensional images—computer-generated pictures utilizing shading techniques to create the appearance of 3D—are sometimes helpful when evaluating facial bone fractures and acetabulum fractures of the hip prior to reconstruction surgery.

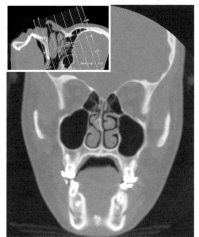

Direct coronal CT of sinuses

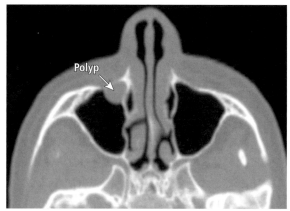

Axial reconstruction of sinuses

Computed Tomography

2.9 What is CTA?

Computed tomography angiography (CTA) is a computer-intensive reconstruction of the vascular structures in the body. Both venous and arterial imaging can be performed using intravenous contrast. Iodinated contrast is delivered through an 18-gauge or larger intravenous catheter. A power injector is used to deliver the contrast. The computer can then subtract away any density that does not contain contrast. The vascular system can be seen in excellent detail. CTA is used to detect thrombosis within veins or arteries, stenosis, aneurysms, and vascular malformations. A common indication is for the detection of pulmonary embolism.

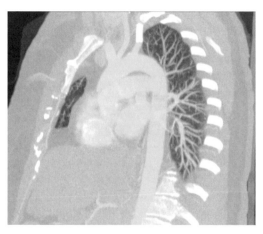

CTA: pulmonary arteries

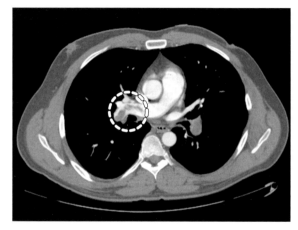

CTA: right pulmonary artery embolus

Computed Tomography

2.10 What are the benefits of CT compared to plain radiography?

CT, by "slicing" the anatomy into thin sections, allows us to look inside the body with fewer overlapping shadows than we get with plain radiography. Because every slice does have a certain thickness and therefore volume, it is possible to be fooled when a section contains parts of two different structures, such as when the top of the diaphragm is included on the lowest images of the lungs. This is called partial volume averaging.

   CT also allows us to quantify radiographic density through measuring Hounsfield units. We can therefore be certain about the composition of a structure or mass. Simple cysts have water density. Lipomas have fat density. Blood, as in intracranial hemorrhage, has a specific range of density. CT is preferred to plain X-rays when more anatomic detail is required, such as for the intracranial structures, sinuses, neck, chest, and abdomen, and for assessing the osseous detail of joints. MRI is preferred for looking at soft tissues such as ligaments, cartilage, and disks.

2.11 What are the benefits of CT compared to MRI?

CT is an excellent modality for looking for intracranial hemorrhage. It remains the first imaging study when intracranial bleeding is suspected (such as hemorrhagic stroke, subdural, epidural, subarachnoid, or intra-parenchymal). CT is excellent for studying cortical bone and is used to assess fracture alignment in the face, cervical spine, acetabulum, knee, and foot (especially the calcaneus). CT continues to be favored in the chest, as well as in the abdomen, although MRI is an excellent modality with many uses in the abdomen. My suggestion is that you consult with the radiologist before ordering an abdominal MRI. CT is generally quicker, less expensive, and more readily available than MRI. It is often better than MRI at assessing cortical bone and for specific density measurements. Please note that there is considerable variation among radiology departments in the type and quality of the imaging equipment; the training, experience, and expertise of the radiologists; and the preferences of the clinical staff. For this reason, expect to find differences in preferred imaging strategies between medical facilities.

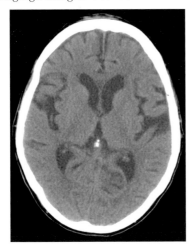

Normal CT (note: skull is white adjacent to brain)

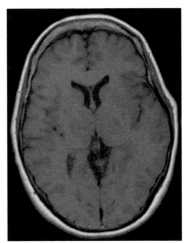

Normal T1 MRI (note: skull is black adjacent to brain)

CHAPTER THREE   ULTRASOUND

3.0 Goals: Understanding how ultrasound works; its uses, strengths, and weaknesses

Objective questions:

3.1 What is ultrasound?
3.2 How does ultrasound work?
3.3 How is an image created with ultrasound?
3.4 When is ultrasound most useful?
3.5 What are the regions of the body and/or diagnoses best imaged with ultrasound?
3.6 What are safety considerations with ultrasound?
3.7 What are 3D and 4D ultrasound?

3.1 What is ultrasound?

Ultrasound is defined as high-frequency sound waves of 20 thousand to 1 million Hz (cycles per second) or greater. (Each peak in a sound wave represents one cycle.) Diagnostic ultrasound operates between 3.5 and 10 million Hz (3.5 and 10 MHz).

3.2 How does ultrasound work?

Ultrasound is created by the high-frequency vibration of a crystal located in the ultrasound transducer, which is a piece of equipment about the size of a small cell phone that fits easily into the hand. The soft, curved end of the transducer is placed on the patient, and gel is used to improve its contact with the skin. During the scanning process, the crystal is stimulated electronically to vibrate. This occurs in an instant, and the crystal then becomes a listening device for the returning echoes from ultrasound reflected back by body tissues. These returning echoes are converted to a gray scale for the creation of an ultrasound image.

Ultrasound

3.3 How is an image created with ultrasound?

As the ultrasound energy travels through tissues of the body, it is scattered, transmitted, or reflected back to the transducer. Ultrasound that is scattered does not help to create an image. Ultrasound that is transmitted produces an echo-free area on the image. Fluid such as ascites, bile within the gallbladder, and serous water within a cyst all appear as sonolucent (echo-free and black on the film) areas on the ultrasound image. Reflected ultrasound creates a density on the ultrasound image (gray or white on the film). The difference in how much ultrasound a given tissue reflects allows us to see individual structures. For example, the pancreas reflects more ultrasound (is more echogenic) than the liver, the liver reflects more than the spleen, and the spleen reflects more than the kidneys.

Important term 1 "Increased through transmission"

When ultrasound passes through a fluid medium, the intensity of the sound energy is not diminished. Therefore, tissues behind the fluid collection are more echogenic (brighter because there is more acoustic power to reflect back to the transducer).

Important term 2 "Posterior acoustical shadowing"

When ultrasound hits a dense object such as a gallstone and is completely reflected, a posterior acoustical shadow is formed. The gallstone is bright and echogenic. Because no ultrasound energy is left to go beyond the stone, an echo void is created, which appears as a wedge-shaped dark area posterior to the dense object.

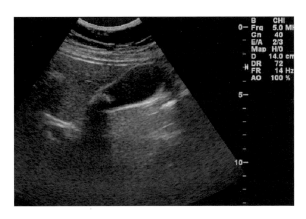

Posterior acoustical shadowing (gallstone)

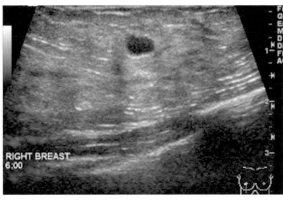

Breast cyst with increase through transmission

Ultrasound

3.4 When is ultrasound most useful?

As a general rule, ultrasound is best at distinguishing the characteristic echo-free appearance seen in fluid collections or cysts. It works best on thin patients and on body parts closest to the skin. Ultrasound does not work well in the presence of gas or air or in larger patients.

3.5 What are the regions of the body and/or diagnoses best imaged with ultrasound?

Appendicitis
Breast
Female pelvis
Gallbladder
Heart
Kidneys
Neonatal brain
Pleural effusion
Pregnancy
Scrotum
Soft tissue masses
Thyroid
Upper abdomen
Vascular structures (venous and arterial)

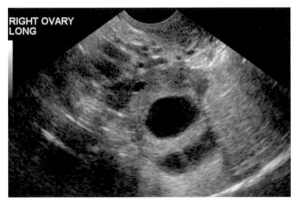

Cyst—right ovary

Solid left breast nodule

Ultrasound

3.6 What are the safety considerations for ultrasound?

Ultrasound is the safest of all current imaging modalities. There is no magnetic field and no radiation to be concerned about. No harmful effects have been proven when ultrasound is performed at diagnostic frequencies.

3.7 What are 3D and 4D ultrasound?

Three-dimensional ultrasound uses the same principles as 2D ultrasound but adds a position-sensing component to produce the effect of a 3D image. As with CT, 3D imaging is helpful to examine contour. Currently, 3D ultrasound is used primarily in pregnancy ultrasound to provide a snapshot of the fetus. The detail possible with 3D ultrasound is incredible, especially in the delicate facial area, but also in the heart chambers and valves. Four-dimensional ultrasound adds the fourth dimension of time. It is essentially a motion video of the three-dimensional fetus. Diaphragm activity, limb movement, and cardiac motion can be seen clearly in real time.

4.0 Goals: Understanding how MRI and PET scanning work: their uses, strengths, and weaknesses

Objective questions:

4.1   How does MRI work?
4.2   What is being imaged with MRI?
4.3   What is meant by "MRI signal"?
4.4   How do I begin to interpret MRI?
4.5   What are the benefits of MRI compared to plain radiography, CT, and ultrasound?
4.6   What are the regions of the body and/or diagnoses best imaged with MRI?
4.7   What are the safety considerations with MRI?
4.8   How does PET scanning work?
4.9   When should a PET scan be requested?
4.10   Are there contraindications to PET scanning?
4.11   What is PET/CT?

MRI / PET

4.1 How does MRI work?

Although it is not critical that the student understand the complex physics of MRI, it does help to have a few very basic concepts in mind when analyzing MR images. The following statements are oversimplifications that I have found helpful. Anyone interested in studying radiology as a vocation is encouraged to learn the true properties and physics in greater detail.

Getting an image from MRI depends upon the presence of protons in the body. Protons are free hydrogen atoms (proton without electrons). They are abundant in the body. With their net positive charge, protons are small magnets, each having a north and a south pole. When placed in a strong magnetic field, enough of these tiny proton magnets align to form a single magnetic vector. A radiofrequency pulse is added to this steady state and tips the net magnetic vector off axis. As the vector returns to its alignment in the magnet, energy is released. It is this energy that is used to create the image.

4.2 What is being imaged with MRI?

In general, MRI is water imaging. Most pathologic conditions in the body are associated with edema, or water formation. MRI is excellent for detecting this water. T1 and T2 are the basic MR imaging sequences (although there are now many more variations in clinical use). With T1, water has no signal and is black. With T2, water has high signal and is white. Proton density (PD) imaging, which is midway between T1 and T2, has some of their advantages. This sequence is very helpful in evaluating the menisci of the knee. For most MRI examinations, two to eight imaging sequences are performed. The faster sequences can be obtained in about two minutes, while more complex sequences can take about 15 minutes. You will hear such terms as *spin echo, fast spin echo, gradient echo, inversion recovery, diffusion weighting, T2*,* and *fat saturation.* Each of these sequences carries advantages and disadvantages. Radiology departments may vary in the MRI imaging sequences they utilize. Most departments follow a manual as a general guideline and make modifications as needed depending on factors such as the strength of the magnet, the pathology being studied, and the preferences of the radiologists.

The terms *open* and *closed magnets* refer to the enclosure that patients are placed in for the examination. Open MRI, in general, provides more room for patient comfort but takes longer because of lower field strength. Closed MRI is more confining but is often faster because it typically has higher field strength. Although debate continues about the relative sharpness and image quality (many believe that the difference between open and closed MRI for most examinations is negligible), either system can provide beautiful diagnostic images of the body.

An MRI machine may use a fixed magnet or a superconducting magnet. A detailed discussion of the differences between the two is beyond the scope of this handbook, but in general a fixed magnet has a lower field strength (lower tesla) and is used in open MRI, while a superconducting magnet has a higher field strenght and is found in most closed MRI units.

Surface coils are important tools for MRI. A surface coil is an antenna that fits closely around the body part to be examined. It increases the radiofrequency signal produced by the body during an MRI.

4.3 What is meant by "MRI signal"?

Whereas in CT and X-ray we use terms such as *density* and *attenuation,* in MRI the term is *signal;* it describes the shades of gray between bright white and black. Describing a white area on MRI, we say that there is high signal. Describing a dark gray or black area, we say that there is low or no signal.

T1 is often referred to as the *anatomy sequence* because water or edema is less conspicuous and anatomy is usually clearly delineated. T2 is known as the *pathologic sequence* because the high signal (white) occurring when there is edema is very easy to see. A good example is effusion in the knee joint. The fluid in the joint is very obvious as white or bright signal on T2-weighted images. Today, there are many variations in MRI imaging sequences, and more are being discovered all the time. These sequences can be used to suppress signal from fat or from free fluid.

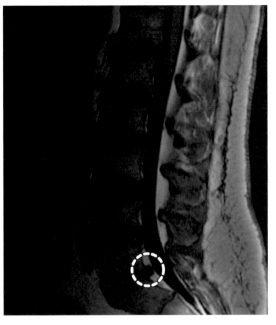

T1 lumbar MRI

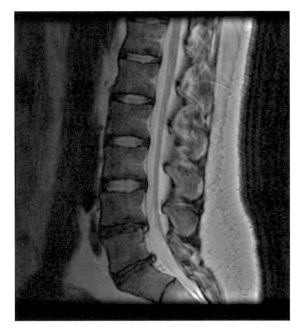

T2 lumbar MRI

MRI / PET

4.4 How do I begin learning to read an MRI?

Begin by learning imaging anatomy. There are many excellent reference texts and Web sites. If you can recognize normal anatomy, pathology becomes easier to detect. If you have access to MRI films, labeling structures with a wax pencil reinforces your learning. Specifically look for normal structures with the signal characteristics of T1 and T2. In other words, when examining an MRI of the brain, first examine the fluid-filled ventricles. The fluid will be black on T1 and white on T2. After mastering imaging anatomy, learn the signal characteristics of normal structures, and finally the signal characteristics of pathologic conditions.

4.5 What are the benefits of MRI compared to plain radiography, CT, and ultrasound?

MRI is a superior imaging modality. No radiation is used, and the anatomic detail it provides is exquisite. The imaging parameters can be varied in multiple ways that continue to evolve, bringing us closer to achieving tissue specificity.

MRI is superior to X-ray and CT in the evaluation of soft tissues such as cartilage, ligaments, soft tissue tumors, fluid collections, neuronal tissue such as the spinal cord, and the white matter tracts of the brain. MRI eliminates overlapping shadows, which are a problem with plain X-rays.

Like CT, MRI uses slices of anatomy that allow us to focus in on specific anatomy and pathology. Unlike CT, MRI can obtain these slices in any imaging plane while the patient remains supine. MRI does not contend with artifacts that can plague CT, such as bone artifacts in the posterior fossa of the brain.

MRI is not limited by bone and air, two limitations of ultrasound.

4.6 What are the regions of the body and/or diagnoses best imaged with MRI?

Abdomen (to clarify CT or ultrasound findings)
Bile ducts and pancreatic duct (magnetic resonance cholangiopancreatography [MRCP])
Brain (especially the posterior fossa, nuclei, cranial nerves, and white matter tracts)
Cervical, thoracic, and lumbar spine
Female pelvis (to clarify ultrasound or CT findings)
Joints
    Elbow
    Fingers
    Foot and ankle
    Hip
    Knee
    Shoulder
    Temporomandibular joint
    Wrist
Staging endometrial cancer
Staging prostate cancer
Vascular structures (magnetic resonance arteriography and venography)

4.7 What are the safety considerations for MRI?

Magnets that are used in diagnostic imaging are strong and potentially dangerous. Most MRI machines operate between 0.3 and 3.0 tesla. The magnetic field of the earth is approximately 1 gauss, or one ten-thousandth of a tesla.

Death and injury have occurred when metal objects became projectiles in a magnetic field. Never enter the MRI scan room with scissors, hemostats, stethoscopes, or anything else that is ferromagnetic. The magnetic strips on credit cards are erased by the magnetic field, pacemakers malfunction, aneurysm clips dislodge, and oxygen tanks can hurtle through the air.

MRI personnel try very hard to screen patients for potential hazards. Never order an MRI without first considering the potential risks to the patient. When in doubt, ask the radiologist or technologist if it is safe for the patient to be scanned. Be particularly careful of pacemakers, metal workers who may have metal shavings in their eyes, and any patient who has had recent surgery. Emergency code situations can occur in the MRI scan room. Stop and think before springing into action. Remember, in an emergency, your first action should be to check your pockets carefully and remove any metal objects before entering the scan room.

> Note: Most postoperative patients can be safely imaged with MRI. Hip-replacement surgery, cholecystectomy, hysterectomy, and many other surgeries do not preclude MRI. The Web site http://MRIsafety.com is a good source for further information.

4.8 How does PET scanning work?

Positron emission tomography (PET) scanning is a branch of nuclear medicine or nuclear imaging, which means that it utilizes radioactive materials to create an image. Nuclear imaging generally depicts physiologic activity and provides less anatomic detail. PET involves the imaging of the metabolic activity of cells within the body. Cancer cells, having rapid and unchecked growth, have much greater metabolic activity than normal cells. When a radioactive substance is tagged to a glucose derivative known as fluorodeoxyglucose (FDG), areas of the body containing such cells can be imaged. When positrons, which are subatomic particles attached to FDG, decay, gamma rays are produced. These rays are detected by a "gamma camera." The image that is created is composed of a background of gamma rays coming from normal cells, reflecting normal metabolic activity, and a highly intense concentration of gamma rays coming from cells with an extremely high metabolic rate—cancer cells.

4.9 When should a PET scan be requested?

Medicare currently covers the following PET indications:

- Evaluation of the solitary pulmonary nodule
- Staging of non-small cell lung cancer
- Detection and localization of recurrent colon cancer
- Staging and characterizing of Hodgkins and non-Hodgkins lymphoma
- Identification of metastatic disease from melanoma
- Diagnosis and staging of esophageal cancer
- Detection of head and neck cancer (excluding CNS and thyroid)
- Restaging of breast cancer and distinguishing of scar from recurrent cancer
- Presurgical evaluation of refractory seizures
- Assessment of myocardial viability
    Source: Medicare press release, http://www.cms.hhs.gov/media/press/release.

The indications for PET continue to expand.

4.10 Are there contraindications to PET scanning?

There are only a few contraindications to PET. Pregnancy is a relative contraindication. Always check with the radiologist before ordering a test that utilizes radiation on a pregnant patient.

4.11 What is PET/CT?

PET/CT is positron emission tomography combined with computed tomography. PET has the advantage of sensitivity for rapidly growing cancer cells, but it provides limited anatomic information. CT is excellent for clearly depicting anatomy, assessing tumor size, and accurately localizing the cancer, and is especially important for evaluating vital structures adjacent to the cancer. But CT cannot detect metabolic activity. PET/CT allows clinicians to see a fused image of physiologic and anatomic information.

CHAPTER FIVE　　CHEST

5.0 Goals: Learning a methodology for interpreting chest radiographs

Objective questions:

- 5.1　What modalities are used to image the chest?
- 5.2　What is PA?
- 5.3　When would I order an AP portable chest?
- 5.4　When would I order an expiratory PA chest?
- 5.5　What does a lateral decubitus chest X-ray show?
- 5.6　I'm looking at the PA and lateral chest. Now what? Where do I start?
- 5.7　How do I examine the mediastinum?
- 5.8　What can I tell about the mediastinum based on density?
- 5.9　How do I examine the hemidiaphragms?
- 5.10　What causes elevation of the diaphragm?
- 5.11　How do I examine the pleura?
- 5.12　What can go wrong in the pleural space?

Chest

5.1 What modalities are used to image the chest?

The most commonly ordered X-ray is a chest X-ray, which is the quickest and most cost-effective way to begin imaging the thorax. Regardless of the diagnosis as it relates to cardiopulmonary disease, a PA and lateral chest X-ray gives valuable information and serves as a baseline to confirm the effectiveness of treatment. An AP chest is done when the patient is unable to be moved, usually because of the severity of his or her illness. As you will learn, the AP portable chest X-ray has definite diagnostic limitations. Sometimes viewing the lungs in expiration is helpful (please see section 5.4). A decubitus chest X-ray takes advantage of gravity. Air goes up and fluid goes down. This maneuver can help us be more specific with a diagnosis. CT, MRI, and PET have specific indications in the thorax, almost always to clarify or further characterize an abnormality seen on the PA and lateral chest X-ray.

Chest imaging modalities:

> PA and lateral chest X-ray
> AP portable chest X-ray
> Expiratory PA chest X-ray
> Lateral decubitus chest X-ray
> Chest CT
> Chest MRI
> PET scanning

5.2 What is PA?

PA stands for *posterior to anterior,* which is the direction of the X-ray beam as it passes through the patient. As the patient stands with the anterior chest wall closest to the film, the technologist asks the patient to take in a deep breath and hold it. X-rays pass from posterior to anterior to expose the film. In this position, the heart is closer to the film than on an AP view and there is less magnification of the cardiac silhouette. For the lateral view, the patient stands with the left side closest to the film, again to reduce magnification of the heart shadow.

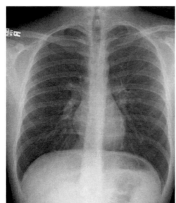

Normal PA chest

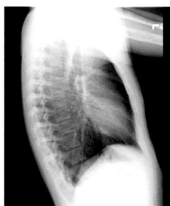

Normal lateral chest

5.3 When would I order an AP portable chest?

If a patient is too unstable or too ill to be transported to the radiology department, the only option is a single view with a portable X-ray machine brought to the bedside. This frequently occurs in the emergency department, in surgery, or in an intensive care unit. An AP portable chest is inferior to a PA or lateral. Problems with an AP chest include the following:

> Magnification of the heart shadow
> Artifacts from lead wires, lines, bedsheets, and skin folds
> Patient motion artifacts
> Patient rotation
> Visualization of the chest in one plane only (a lateral is not performed mobile)
> Variable exposure factors related to the equipment used

5.4 When would I order an expiratory PA chest?

The two most common indications for an expiratory PA chest are pneumothorax and foreign body aspiration. An expiratory phase film helps with the following:

> **Suspected pneumothorax:** Forcing air out of the lungs allows the visceral pleura and the air in the pleural space to be observed to greater advantage. When the air inside the lung is forced out by expiration, the density of the lung increases. The air trapped in the pleural space remains low in density (air density shows as black). The trapped air in the pneumothorax then becomes easier to identify.

Suspected foreign body: If a patient, usually a child, aspirates a foreign body, it will commonly lodge in the right main stem bronchus. There it may act as a ball valve, allowing air to pass into the lung but not out. An expiratory film will demonstrate the persistent aeration of the obstructed lung, even if the foreign body is not opaque (visible). The obstructed lung will stay inflated on both inspiration and expiration, while the unaffected lung will inflate and empty.

5.5 What does a lateral decubitus chest X-ray show?

We often use gravity to help us differentiate between free-flowing pleural effusion and loculated fluid (fluid caught up in an area of pleural scarring) or pleural thickening. A transudate is a thin fluid collection that layers in the pleural space along the lateral thoracic wall when the affected side is down. The lateral decubitus film helps to demonstrate that the fluid is freely movable. We can thus better estimate the quantity of fluid and plan for thoracentesis (drawing off fluid for diagnosis or therapy). An exudate is a thick or viscous fluid collection. Exudates may be seen in infection (pyothorax) or in association with cancer (mesothelioma or metastatic disease). Exudates are slower to layer on a decubitus X-ray and may not layer at all.

TEST YOUR KNOWLEDGE:

You suspect a freely movable right pleural effusion (transudate). What X-ray study would you request?

Answer: PA and lateral chest with a right lateral decubitus view.

Chest

5.6 I'm looking at the PA and lateral chest. Now what? Where do I start?

1. Check the name and the date on the radiograph.

2. Examine the film for quality. Is it over- or underexposed? If you can see the disk spaces in the thoracic spine through the heart shadow on a PA radiograph, the film is overexposed. Is the patient rotated? Is there a good depth of inspiration? If you can count 8.5–11 posterior rib structures above the diaphragm, that's a good inspiration.

3. Use the mnemonic "MDPLOTS" as a guide:
   - **M** = Mediastinum
   - **D** = Diaphragm
   - **P** = Pleura
   - **L** = Lungs
   - **O** = Osseous structures
   - **T** = Trachea
   - **S** = Soft tissues

KEY POINT:

Any structure, normal or pathologic, should be analyzed for

1. Size	3. Position
2. Shape and contour	4. Density

5.7 How do I examine the mediastinum?

The boundaries of the mediastinum are noted below. If you understand what structures live there, you will understand what pathologies can occur there. The mediastinum has normal and predictable contours, and evaluating the mediastinum on a chest X-ray requires contour assessment.

On the PA view, superiorly, the right and left lateral margins of the mediastinum are slightly concave. The right border is created by the superior vena cava and the left border is created by the left subclavian artery. The trachea should be midline, except at the level of the aortic arch where the trachea descends to the right. As we move caudally, we will see a contour bulge on the left created by the aortic arch. A concavity called the aorticopulmonary window normally occurs between the undersurface of the aortic arch and the top of the left main pulmonary artery. On the right is a normal contour bulge where the azygos vein enters the superior vena cava. The hilar areas are located along both sides of the heart shadow. The vessels should resemble the branching of a tree trunk: three major branches on the right and two on the left. The pulmonary veins also enter the mediastinum at this location. Therefore, the hilar areas are a busy place and require close scrutiny on the radiograph. The ascending aorta can cause a normal, smooth convexity just above the right hilum leading to the aortic arch. On the left, there may be a subtle contour bulge made by the left atrium. The right heart border is created by the right atrium. The left heart border is created by a small segment of the left atrium but predominantly the left ventricle.

Chest

Divisions of the mediastinum:

1. Superior mediastinum: Contents of the chest above a line drawn between T5 and the sternal manubrium, fat, small lymph nodes, arteries, veins, and sometimes the thyroid gland.
2. Inferior mediastinum:
   a. Anterior: The anterior boundary of the anterior part is the posterior sternum. Its posterior boundary is the pericardium of the heart. It contains fat, small lymph nodes, and the thymus gland.
   b. Middle: The middle mediastinum is composed of the pericardium and the heart.
   c. Posterior: The anterior boundary of the posterior mediastinum is the posterior pericardial sac. The posterior boundary is the anterior surfaces of the bodies of thoracic vertebrae T5–T12. Neural tissue, the esophagus, and lymph nodes live here.

Summary of mediastinal evaluation:

1. The *width* of the mediastinum
2. The shape or *contour*
3. The *midline position* of the mediastinal structures
4. The *density* of the mediastinum (i.e., calcium density in mediastinal teratoma)

Common causes of abnormally widened superior mediastinum:

1. Distention of the superior vena cava in CHF
2. Mediastinal hemorrhage following blunt chest trauma
3. Aneurysm of any of the three aortic arch branches (brachiocephalic, left common carotid, and left subclavian arteries)
4. Excessive mediastinal fat (Cushing's disease, steroid use)
5. Lymphadenopathy
6. Metastatic disease
7. Tumors such as thymoma, teratoma, or substernal goiter
8. Air (pneumomediastinum)

Causes of widened superior mediastinum with smooth contours:

1. Distension of the superior vena cava
2. Hemorrhage
3. Fat

Chest

Causes of lobulated superior mediastinal contour:

1. Aneurysms
2. Masses
3. Lymphadenopathy

Causes of shift of the mediastinum:

1. Toward pathology: volume loss (atelectasis), postoperative lobectomy or pneumonectomy, scarring or fibrosis
2. Away from pathology: lung mass, tension pneumothorax, large pleural effusion, pulmonary consolidation (rare)

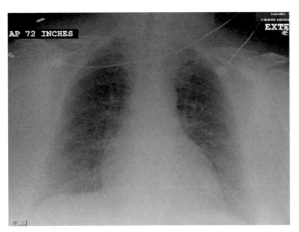

Chest X-ray: left superior mediastinal mass

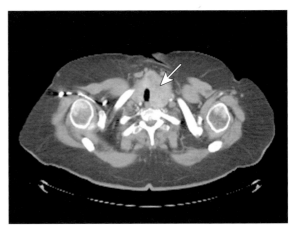

CT: thyroid mass

Chest

5.8 What can I tell about the mediastinum based on density?

Calcification is the most helpful density to identify when looking at the mediastinum. Calcium density can be seen in

Teratomas
Granulomatous lymph nodes (histoplasmosis)
Calcified walls of an aneurysm
Goiters (rare)

5.9 How do I examine the hemidiaphragms?

Analyzing the hemidiaphragms involves primarily assessing diaphragmatic position and contour. The right hemidiaphragm is usually higher than the left, probably because of the liver being below the right hemidiaphragm and the heart being above the left hemidiaphragm. If specific information about diaphragmatic motion is required, ask for chest fluoroscopy. The radiologist can watch the hemidiaphragms move during expiration, inspiration, sniffing, and Valsalva maneuvers.

5.10 What causes elevation of the diaphragm?

The diaphragm can be pushed or pulled. What can push the diaphragm down?

> Pressure buildup in the pleural space in tension pneumothorax
> Large pleural effusions
> Air trapping in the lungs, such as with emphysema or asthma
> Tumors, pleural and pulmonary
> Consolidating pneumonia or lung abscess

What can push the diaphragm up?

> Hepatic enlargement
> Ascites
> Splenomegaly
> Air buildup in the hepatic flexure, transverse colon, or splenic flexure

What can pull the diaphragm up?

> Scar tissue in a lower lobe of the lung
> Atelectasis in a lower lobe
> Previous pneumonectomy or lobectomy; with loss of volume, the diaphragm rises to fill the void
>
> Note: Masses arising from the diaphragm itself are rare.

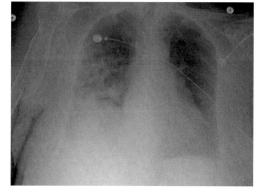

Elevated right diaphragm consistent
with RLL volume loss

Chest

5.11 How do I examine the pleura?

The pleural space is actually a potential space between the parietal pleura, which lines the inside of the chest wall and the visceral pleura, which covers the lungs. A small amount of fluid and a slight negative pressure keep the pleural linings together. When examining the pleura, begin at the medial aspect of the right diaphragm, follow the diaphragm laterally, examine the lateral chest wall from bottom to top, and continue down the mediastinum to the point where you began. Repeat the process on the left side. If the pleura is visible, it is abnormal.

5.12 What can go wrong in the pleural space?

Typically, what can go wrong in the pleural space is that something else fills it, such as

Air in the case of pneumothorax
Lymph in chylothorax
Pus (pathogens and inflammatory cells) in empyema
Serous (thin) fluid in pleural effusion
Exudative (thick) fluid in pleural effusion
Cancer cells in malignant effusion
Blood in hemothorax
Scar tissue (pleural thickening) in diseases such as asbestosis and tuberculosis

The two most common conditions resulting in an abnormal pleural space are pneumothorax and serous pleural effusion.

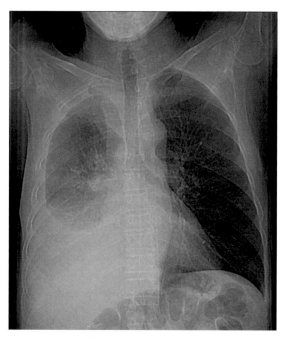

Right pleural effusion

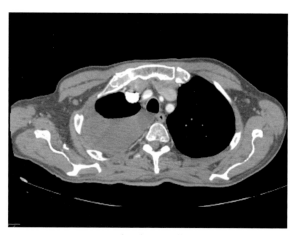

CT: right pleural effusion

Chest

5.13 How can I recognize a pneumothorax on a chest X-ray?

If you carefully examine the most gravity-independent portion of the chest (the apices on an upright PA radiograph), you will note that the lung markings (composed of blood vessels and bronchial structures) do not extend all the way to the chest wall. You will be able to see the thin visceral pleura. The abnormally accumulated air in the pleural space is clear and devoid of any markings. To exaggerate this appearance, request an expiratory phase PA chest X-ray, which is taken with the patient at end exhalation. The markings in the lungs become accentuated in expiration, and therefore the density difference between the partially empty lung tissue and the air in the pleural space becomes more obvious.

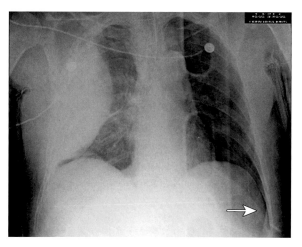

Deep sulcus sign (left pneumothorax)/right hemothorax

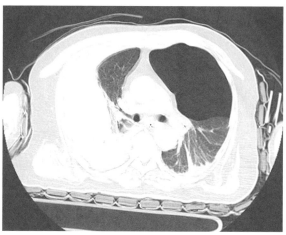

Right hemothorax/left pneumothorax on CT

Chest

5.14 What does pleural effusion look like?

Fluid falls to fill the most gravity-dependent portion of the pleural space. This occurs adjacent to the diaphragms in the posterior and lateral costophrenic angles. The costophrenic angles are the key to the diagnosis. The apex of the sharp angle between the chest wall and the diaphragm should be pointing down. When this space fills with fluid, the angles are filled in (blunted). Fluid clinging to the edges of the costophrenic angle creates a meniscus (cup shape).

A useful maneuver to determine if the fluid is serous and free to flow in the pleural space is to place the patient on his or her side with the effusion side down. The chest X-ray will show the fluid layering along the lateral chest wall. Doing this will provide two important pieces of information: first, you will know that the fluid is thin enough to move, and second, you will know that it is not loculated or trapped. A film can be obtained with the patient lying in a lateral decubitus position, that is, on his or her side. If you suspect a right pleural effusion, order a right lateral decubitus chest X-ray.

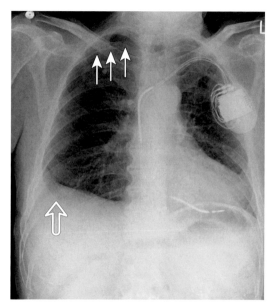

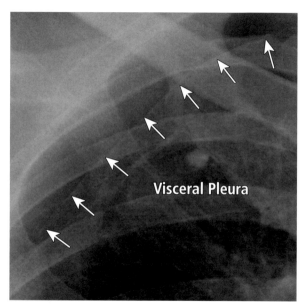

Arrows: right apical pneumothorax
Block arrow: pleural effusion

Visible visceral pleura = pneumothorax

Chest

5.15 How do I examine the lungs?

The lungs are most often the primary reason for obtaining a chest X-ray. The right side of the chest should be compared to the left side from top to bottom. I like to compare the top thirds of the lungs first, then the middle thirds, and finally the bottom thirds. As always, a global or overall impression of both lungs helps to give an initial impression. Pathology in the lungs can be broken down into conditions that fill the lungs and those that collapse the lungs.

5.16 What things can fill the lungs?

Excessive air, such as with emphysema or asthma
Blood, pus, or fluid in the alveolar spaces
Thickened connective tissue (the interstitial portions) of the lungs
Tumors

5.17 What are the findings in emphysema?

Emphysema and asthma are common forms of chronic obstructive pulmonary disease. Air gets into the alveolar spaces but has trouble getting out because of chronic inflammatory narrowing, spasm, or mucus within the bronchi. Because air is black on an X-ray, when there is excess air, the lungs look darker than normal (hyperlucent). As the chest accommodates more volume, the anterior to posterior diameter increases (barrel chest) and the space behind the sternum widens (increased retrosternal clear space). You may notice that the rib spaces are wider and the diaphragms, normally convex superiorly, are flattened or depressed. Pressure from the increased air volume compresses the peripheral veins such that the pulmonary vasculature appears tapered. The heart also has to pump against this increased pressure, resulting in enlargement of the central pulmonary arteries with peripheral arterial narrowing.

Summary of findings in chronic obstructive pulmonary disease:

> Pulmonary overaeration (dark-looking lungs)
> Increased AP diameter of the chest
> Widened retrosternal clear space
> Widened intercostal spaces
> Flattening of the hemidiaphragms
> Tapering of the peripheral pulmonary
>   vasculature
> Engorgement of the central pulmonary
>   arteries

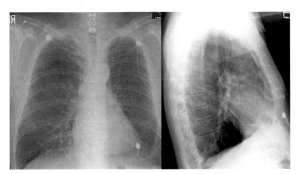

Chronic obstructive pulmonary disease

Chest

5.18 What are the causes of alveolar lung disease?

In the pure form of alveolar lung disease (also called air space disease), fluid of some type is occupying the air sacs. The three types of fluid responsible for the vast majority of alveolar lung disease are pus (pneumonia), water (pulmonary edema), and blood (pulmonary hemorrhage). On a chest X-ray, alveolar lung disease appears as a cumulus cloud. The opacity is coalescent and can vary in density from wispy to dense. *Consolidation* is the term applied to the densest type of alveolar lung disease. The air bronchogram is the hallmark of alveolar lung disease. This important sign occurs when the alveolar sacs within the acini of the lung fill with blood, pus, or fluid, allowing us to see the air-filled bronchi. Without alveolar disease, the bronchi are not visible because the alveoli and the adjacent bronchi are filled with air and cannot be distinguished from one another.

Summary: Causes of alveolar lung disease

> Blood = Pulmonary laceration, contusion, Goodpasture's syndrome
> Pus = Any pneumonia, but especially bacterial pneumonia
> Fluid = Pulmonary edema from any cause, congestive heart failure, near-drowning, high-altitude pulmonary edema

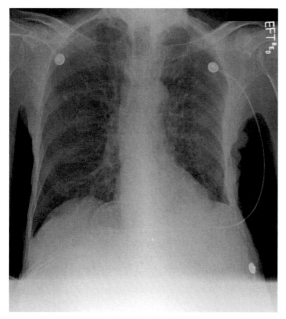

Chest X-ray: prepneumonia

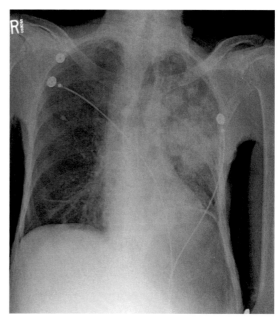

Left upper lobe pneumonia

Chest

5.19 What is interstitial lung disease?

Interstitial lung disease encompasses a large number of pathologic conditions. The interstitium of the lung is the connective tissue support structure and the lymphatics, which make up a network of linear and web-like tissues akin to the highways, streets, and alleys of a city. When these structures become congested with fluid, tumor cells, or inflammatory cells, or when they become overgrown and thickened, they show up on a chest X-ray as thickened linear or weblike opacities or small nodular opacities. Interstitial lung disease can be reticular (all linear), nodular (all small nodular opacities), or reticulonodular (both).

Mnemonic for interstitial lung disease: "CAT HIDES"

C = Collagen vascular diseases
A = Arthritis (rheumatoid lung, ankylosing spondylitis)
T = Tuberculosis
H = Hemosiderosis
I = Infection (TB, fungal or viral), Irradiation treatment
D = Drug-induced
E = Eosinophilic granuloma, Edema
S = Sarcoidosis, Scleroderma

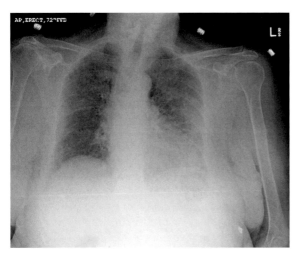

Interstitial pneumonia

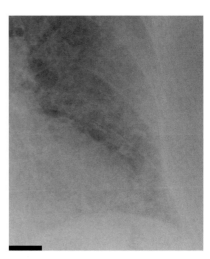

Close-up: interstitial disease

Chest

5.20 What are the findings in congestive heart failure (CHF)?

Cardiac enlargement with a cardiac-to-thoracic (C/T) ratio of 0.50 or greater is often seen in left heart failure. A subtle finding in early congestive heart failure is engorgement of the upper lobe pulmonary veins. This is called *cephalization* in reference to the upper lobe venous congestion. The mediastinum may appear widened due to engorgement of the superior vena cava (widening of the vascular pedicle). Kerley B lines are small linear opacities that typically occur in the lateral aspect of the lower lobes at right angles to the pleura. These thin, approximately 2 cm-long opacities represent perilymphatic fluid resulting from volume overload. Eventually, fluid can distend the interstitial lung structures (interstitial pulmonary edema) and/or the alveolar spaces (alveolar pulmonary edema). As CHF progresses, there is often increasing bilateral pleural effusion.

Summary of findings in CHF:

Cardiac enlargement (C/T ratio of 0.50 or greater)
Cephalization
Widening of the vascular pedicle
Kerley B lines
Interstitial and/or alveolar pulmonary edema
Bilateral pleural effusion

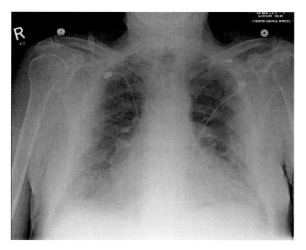

Congestive heart failure

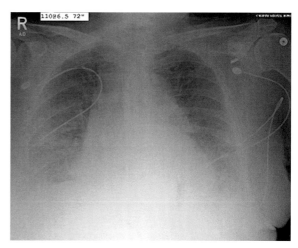

Moderate congestive heart failure

Chest

5.21 How do I examine the osseous structures of the thorax?

The only way to do a complete assessment of bones is to examine them one by one. Start with the right shoulder, examine the right clavicle, the right ribs, the cervical spine and mandible, the left clavicle, the left shoulder, the left ribs, and finally the thoracic spine. You will be looking for signs of osseous destruction or fracture.

5.22 How do I examine the trachea?

The trachea is usually easy to see. It should be midline except where it deviates to the right at the level of the aortic arch. Because neck and mediastinal masses often displace the trachea, it is important to examine the trachea for position. There are also a few abnormalities relating to tracheal size. Weakening of the tracheal cartilage can result in a dilated trachea. Chronic inflammation, trauma, or infection can cause tracheal stenosis (narrowing).

5.23 How do I examine the visible soft tissues of the thorax and upper abdomen?

Start with the stomach bubble. Because all of us have at least some air in our stomachs, the stomach bubble is a constant finding in the left upper quadrant. If the bubble is displaced medially or toward the right side, consider splenomegaly or splenic hematoma. If the bubble is overly distended, consider bowel obstruction. After checking the stomach, scan all of the other visible soft tissues in a clockwise fashion. You will be looking for signs of mass, opaque foreign bodies, evidence of previous surgery, and areas of asymmetry that may reflect swelling or tumors. Your last stop is beneath the hemidiaphragms, where you will specifically look for free air in the abdomen. You will most likely see it on the right side because the right diaphragm is higher than the left and the liver serves as a solid background of density for comparison of air density to soft tissue density.

5.24 How do I evaluate tubes and lines on a chest X-ray?

An endotracheal tube should terminate at the top of the aortic arch. This will be at approximately the T4 level and will place the end of the tube about 4 cm above the carina. Placement below this level raises the risk that the tube could enter the right or left main stem bronchus (usually the right because it is a straighter shot). If this happens, the opposite lung may collapse and the lung on the affected side may become hyperinflated, leading to pneumothorax and/or pneumomediastinum. Placement above the T2 level raises the risk of inflating the balloon cuff too high.

Chest tubes are used to remove something from the pleural space. In the case of pneumothorax, the chest tube is on suction to remove air from the pleural space. In this instance the tube should be in the most gravity-independent position, the apical region of the chest. If the tube is placed to remove blood, pus, or fluid, it should be in the most gravity-dependent area of the chest, posterior and inferior in the thorax. If the fluid is loculated in a different area, the chest tube should be placed in the most gravity-dependent part of the collection.

Chest

5.25 When would I order a chest CT?

CT is generally the imaging procedure of choice after chest X-ray. CT provides excellent anatomic detail of the mediastinum, hemidiaphragms, pleura, lungs, osseous structures, trachea, and soft tissues.

VITAMINS D and C mnemonic for general medical differential diagnosis:

> **V** = Vascular diseases:
>
>> Suspected pulmonary embolism (order as computed tomography angiogram [CTA])
>> Suspected thoracic aortic aneurysm, dissection, or coarctation
>> Anomalous pulmonary venous return
>
> **I** = Infection, Inflammation, Inhalation disease:
>
>> Lung abscess
>> Pyothorax (infection in the pleural space)
>> Refinement of the differential diagnosis in interstitial lung disease
>
> **T** = Trauma:
>
>> Pulmonary laceration
>> Aortic disruption
>> Traumatic esophageal rupture
>
> **A** = Allergic or Autoimmune disease:
>
>> Rheumatoid lung
>> Bronchiolitis obliterans

M = Metabolic disease:

Substernal goiter

I = Idiopathic disease:

Sarcoidosis

N = Neoplasia:

Evaluation of pulmonary nodule(s)
Evaluation of a pulmonary mass (defined as a nodule 3 cm or larger)
Metastatic disease
Mediastinal mass (teratoma, lymphoma, neurogenic tumors, thymoma)

D = Developmental:

Pulmonary sequestration
Diaphragmatic hernia

C = Cardiac:

Left ventricular aneurysm
Valvular calcification
Coronary calcium scoring
Coronary CTA

Chest

5.26 What are the indications for chest MRI?

MRI is a modality best saved for specialized situations. The heart and great vessels can also be studied to great advantage. Because CT is effective, quick, and readily available, I suggest before requesting an MRI of the chest, you first check with the radiologist. Doing so will dramatically improve information sharing and facilitate the best use of resources for arriving at the correct diagnosis.

5.27 When would I order a PET scan of the chest?

Indications for PET imaging:

Evaluation of a focal pulmonary abnormality, as in diagnosis of a solitary pulmonary nodule (SPN)
Preoperative staging for bronchogenic carcinoma, which includes mediastinal and hilar staging as well as extrathoracic staging
Staging of recurrent tumor

5.28 How can I distinguish bacterial from viral pneumonia?

In general, bacterial pneumonia produces air space (alveolar) lung opacities while viral pneumonia produces interstitial lung disease.

Bacterial pneumonia often presents with alveolar opacity confined to a lobe or segment of a lobe. Pneumococcal pneumonia is the pathogen most frequently associated with lobar alveolar disease. Klebsiella pneumonia is often associated with alveolar disease that produces bowing of adjacent fissures. Staphylococcal pneumonia can be very aggressive, presenting with dense consolidation that is not stopped by fissures. Staphylococcal pneumonia tends to create cavities (abscesses) and is a common cause of empyema.

Viral pneumonia is more common in children but can occur in any age group. Occasionally there is associated hilar lymph node enlargement. A common finding in viral infections is peribronchial thickening (thickening of the bronchial wall). Peribronchial thickening is easiest to recognize when a bronchus is viewed end on. Fungal pneumonia may produce interstitial lung disease, alveolar disease, or a combination of both. Fungi are a common cause of cystic cavitation in the lungs.

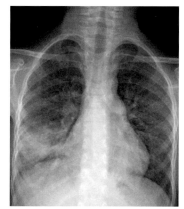

Bacterial pneumonia

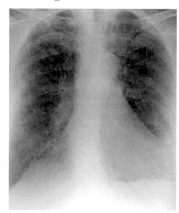

Viral pneumonia

Chest

5.29 How will I recognize lung cancer?

Lung cancer can present on a chest X-ray in multiple ways. Any nodule or mass within the lung that is non-calcified must be considered possible lung cancer. A solitary density is considered to be a nodule if it is smaller than 3 cm and a mass if it is larger than 3 cm. Biopsy is the only definitive means for confirming cancer. If the nodule is over 1 cm, a PET scan can help determine whether the nodule requires biopsy. Increased metabolic activity of a nodule on the PET scan would prompt a biopsy, while a negative PET scan would lead to imaging surveillance. Nodules less than 1 cm are most often followed by surveillance, unless there is strong suspicion of malignancy based on imaging appearance (stellate margins) or clinical grounds.

Surveillance of lung nodules is most often completed with chest X-ray and chest CT performed at 3, 6, 12, and 24 months following the discovery of the nodule. If the nodule has remained stable for 2 years, the chance of malignancy is slim.

Imaging characteristics of a malignant lung nodule include irregular or stellate margins, lack of calcification, increasing size from previous examinations, and lymphadenopathy. Multiple noncalcified lesions, even if they are smoothly marginated, strongly suggest metastatic disease. Lung cancer can often present as pneumonia. Before the patient is deemed healthy, it is important that follow-up chest X-rays document complete resolution of pneumonia. A pulmonary malignancy may produce bronchial obstruction, leading to pneumonia and often slow or incomplete resolution of the resulting air space disease. For the same reason, malignancy can present as an area of atelectasis or volume loss in lungs. In these cases, if volume loss does not resolve over a period of two to four weeks, CT and/or bronchoscopy should be considered.

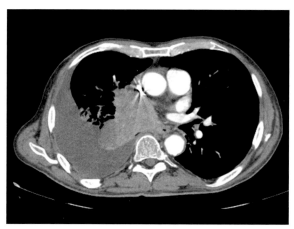

CT: lung cancer

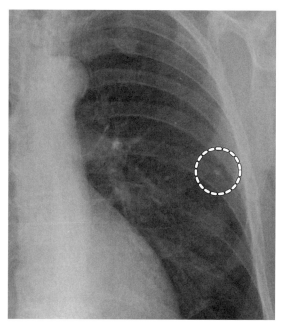

Calcified granuloma

CHAPTER SIX — ABDOMINAL

6.0 Goals: Learning a methodology for interpreting abdominal radiographs

Objective questions:

6.1 How can I systematically analyze an abdominal X-ray?
6.2 What does small bowel obstruction look like?
6.3 What does colon obstruction look like?
6.4 How can I identify free intraperitoneal air?
6.5 What are common causes of pneumoperitoneum?
6.6 What is an acute abdominal series?
6.7 How is CT used in abdominal imaging?
6.8 When is ultrasound appropriate in the abdomen?
6.9 Is MRI useful in abdominal imaging?

6.1 How can I systematically analyze an abdominal X-ray?

I recommend using the five basic radiographic densities as a pattern approach.

Air: Air is normally present in small amounts throughout the intestine, from the stomach to the rectum. Too much air in the intestine can be seen in obstruction and hypodynamic ileus. Sometimes air is seen outside of the bowel. This can be caused by bowel perforation, such as a gastric or duodenal ulcer or a ruptured colon diverticulum. Air can also be seen in the peritoneal cavity after abdominal surgery.

Fat: Several fat stripes are visible on an abdominal radiograph. The properitoneal fat stripe is often visible between the abdominal musculature and the colon. It is situated between the parietal peritoneum and the abdominal wall (seen laterally on AP view). Increased distance between the properitoneal fat stripe and the colon is seen in ascites. The psoas muscles also have a companion fat stripe that should be examined for symmetry. If the psoas fat stripe is absent on one side, consider an overlying inflammatory process (i.e., loss of the right psoas fat stripe in appendicitis).

Soft tissue/fluid: Soft tissue density consists of masses and the major solid organs. The liver, spleen, kidneys, and urinary bladder are the organs most likely to be seen on an abdominal film. Not only are these the largest organs, but they are also surrounded by fat and therefore can often be discerned. Other organs may become visible if they contain calcifications, such as pancreatic calcifications seen in chronic pancreatitis. Look for each solid organ on the abdominal radiograph, checking for enlargement (organomegaly) or mass. Fluid presents in the abdomen as hazy, ground-glass density. In ascites, bowel loops are pushed to the central abdomen (increased distance may be noted between the properitoneal fat stripe and the colon).

Abdomen

Mineral: There are many pathologic conditions in the abdomen associated with calcification:

- Gallstones
- Calcified gallbladder wall (porcelain gallbladder, increased incidence of carcinoma)
- Kidney, ureteral, or bladder stones
- Pancreatic calcifications (chronic pancreatitis)
- Vascular calcification
- Splenic or hepatic calcified granulomatous disease
- Adrenal calcification (usually seen after adrenal hemorrhage)
- Appendicolith

In addition, the skeleton is mineral density that requires review. A search should be made for fractures, metastatic disease, and all other pathologic conditions affecting bone.

Metal: A search for metal density is the final step in the review of the abdomen X-ray. There are no natural metallic densities in the body. The following is a partial list of metal that may be found on an abdominal radiograph:

- Bullets, BBs, pellets
- Foreign bodies
- Surgical clips
- Recent dental work (swallowed dental amalgam)
- Swallowed objects (most often coins)
- Artifacts (snaps, lead wires, objects remaining in clothing pockets)

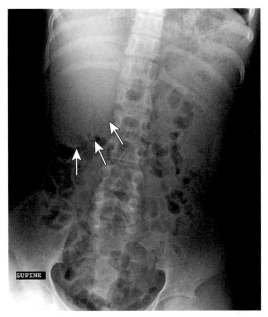

Hepatomegaly

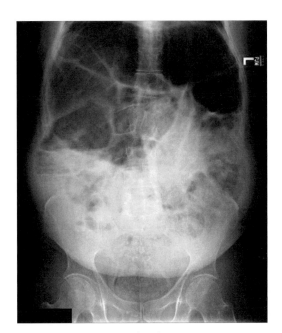

Colon ileus

Abdomen

6.2 What does small bowel obstruction look like?

Small bowel obstruction is most often caused by postsurgical scar tissue (adhesions), but there are many other possible causes, such as tumor, foreign body, internal hernias, and external compression. Regardless of the cause, in a complete small bowel obstruction, air progressively builds up proximal to the obstruction and diminishes past the obstruction. The small bowel normally measures less than 3 cm in diameter. In obstruction, the bowel reaches and may exceed 3 cm in diameter as air builds up proximal to the obstruction. The intestine maintains a state of hypertonicity, resulting in the high-pitched active bowel sounds that are heard clinically. As fluid is propelled further in the small bowel, it too reaches the point of obstruction, creating an important radiographic sign: asynchronous air-fluid leveling (fluid leveling of unequal heights in the same bowel loop), or a "stair-step" pattern. This pattern is seen only on erect or decubitus X-rays. A fluid level is the density interface caused by fluid sinking to the gravity-dependent areas and air rising above the fluid.

Summary of findings in small bowel obstruction:

   Air-distended small bowel to 3 cm or greater
   Diminished or absent colon and rectal gas
   Asynchronous air-fluid leveling (stair-step pattern)

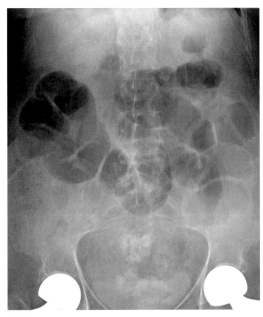

Small bowel obstruction

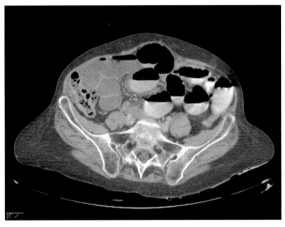

CT scan: small bowel obstruction

6.3 What does colon obstruction look like?

Colon obstruction may be caused by postsurgical adhesions, tumors, inflammatory conditions such as diverticulitis, hernias, and twisting of the bowel (volvulus) among other etiologies. Because the colon is larger than the small bowel, it can distend much further, sometimes reaching 12 cm or more. Air continuously builds proximal to the obstruction and is expelled distal to the obstruction. The result is air-distended small bowel and colon to the site of the obstruction. Upright filming demonstrates air-fluid leveling, but the stair-step pattern is less pronounced or absent due to the large caliber and distensibility of the colon. In volvulus, the colon twists around an unusually long mesentery. Sigmoid volvulus presents with the shape of a coffee bean.

Summary of findings in colon obstruction:

Gas-distended colon loops that may exceed 12 cm
Little or no air distal to the obstruction
Air-fluid levels with little or no stair-step pattern
Coffee-bean sign in sigmoid volvulus

6.4 How can I identify free intraperitoneal air (pneumoperitoneum)?

In radiology, we frequently use the effects of gravity to help us make a diagnosis. A great example is when we search for pneumoperitoneum. Common causes of pneumoperitoneum include recent abdominal surgery, ruptured colon diverticulum, and perforated ulcer. The best way to look for free air is with the patient sitting upright for a period of 5 to 10 minutes. Air percolates around the abdominal viscera, rising to the most gravity-independent site beneath the right diaphragm. If the patient is too unstable to sit upright, a left decubitus abdominal X-ray should be performed. In this position, the left side of the patient is down and the right side is up. Free air will collect beneath the right lateral abdominal wall. The liver serves as a good density background for recognizing the free air.

Detecting free air in the supine position is much more difficult. If there is a lot of free air, we may be able to see both sides of the bowel wall (Rigler's sign). The football sign is another possible, albeit uncommon, indicator of free air. It is caused by air collecting in the shape of a football in the right upper quadrant on both sides of the falciform ligament.

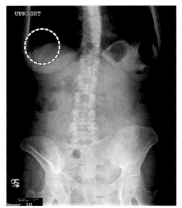

Pneumoperitoneum

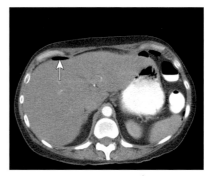

Free air anterior to liver

Abdomen

6.5 What are common causes of pneumoperitoneum?

Recent abdominal surgery, open or laproscopic, always results in at least a small amount of free air. This air is slowly absorbed into the bloodstream. Delayed pneumoperitoneum can last several weeks (there has been a report of residual air eight weeks after surgery). With no history of surgery, a ruptured colon diverticulum and a perforated gastric or duodenal ulcer are the most common causes of pneumoperitoneum. Air can be introduced into the peritoneal cavity through trauma or iatrogenic means, such as viscus perforation during endoscopy.

6.6 What is an acute abdominal series?

An acute abdominal series is one of the most common X-ray requests made in the emergency department. Three views are obtained: a supine abdominal film, an erect or left lateral decubitus abdominal film, and a PA chest X-ray. The supine abdomen is used to assess the intestinal gas pattern, look for organ enlargement or mass, search for pathologic calcifications such as kidney stones, and rule out opaque foreign bodies. The erect abdominal film must include both diaphragms. Free intraperitoneal air will rise to the area beneath the diaphragms. The erect film also allows for the assessment of air-fluid levels in the bowel. Synchronous air-fluid levels are seen in hypodynamic ileus, while asynchronous air-fluid levels are seen in dynamic ileus (obstruction). The PA chest X-ray gives you one more chance to evaluate for air under the diaphragms, but it is primarily used to look for chest causes of abdominal pain, such as lower lobe pneumonia. Some abdominal conditions, such as pancreatitis, will present with pleural effusion, which is best seen on the chest X-ray.

Films obtained in an acute abdominal series:

Supine abdominal X-ray
Erect or left lateral decubitus abdominal X-ray
PA chest

Abdomen

6.7 How is CT used in abdominal imaging?

CT is the procedure of choice for nearly any abdominal condition, with the exception of gallbladder pathology, for which ultrasound is superior. Common reasons to request an abdominal CT are pain, suspected mass pathology, and metastasis. Reasons to order an abdominal CT include the following:

- Abdominal aortic aneurysm
- Abdominal metastatic disease
- Abdominal trauma (lacerated spleen, liver, or kidney)
- Adrenal masses
- Appendicitis
- Cirrhosis
- Diverticulitis
- Gallbladder abscess (phlegmon)
- Hepatic metastatic disease
- Inflammatory bowel disease
- Pancreatic cancer
- Pancreatitis (acute, subacute, or chronic)
- Renal calculus disease
- Renal mass (benign or malignant)

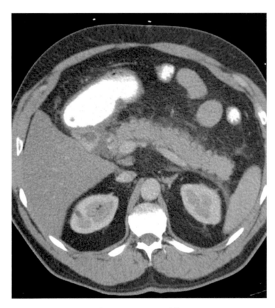

Acute pancreatitis

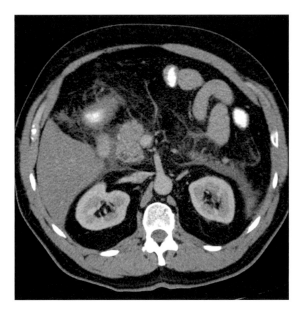

Inflammatory changes; mesenteric fat

Abdomen

6.8 When is ultrasound appropriate in the abdomen?

Ultrasound is best for vascular structures, fluid-filled structures, the female pelvis, and the scrotum. It is generally best for fluid imaging. Ultrasound uses no radiation, can be performed regardless of organ failure, and is readily available. Large patients and patients with gaseous distention of bowel are poor candidates for ultrasound because air tends to scatter the sound rather than conducting it or reflecting it back to the transducer. Reasons to order an abdominal ultrasound include the following:

Gallstones and other gallbladder disease
Abdominal aortic aneurysm
Appendicitis (especially in children)
Pyloric stenosis
Renal cyst
Renal obstruction

6.9 Is MRI useful in abdominal imaging?

MRI adds an additional set of imaging characteristics to the evaluation of any type of pathology. For example, MRI can help differentiate hepatic hemangioma from hepatic adenoma or other tumor. Because MRI can reveal information about the water content, lipid content, and tissue vascularity of a structure, we can use this information to refine the differential diagnosis or make a specific diagnosis. Usually, when multiple imaging modalities are combined, the information obtained leads to a more specific diagnosis. A great example is an adrenal mass. Because 70% of benign adrenal adenomas contain lipid, and because MRI can demonstrate lipid signal characteristics, a specific diagnosis is made possible. Abdominal MRI is generally used to clarify an existing imaging finding from another modality by adding information about tissue characteristics. Reasons to order an abdominal MRI include the following:

Hepatic hemangioma
Other hepatic tumors that continue to have an unclear diagnosis on CT or ultrasound
Bile duct dilatation (magnetic resonance cholangiopancreatography [MRCP])
Arterial pathology (magnetic resonance angiography [MRA])
Staging endometrial cancer
Staging prostate cancer

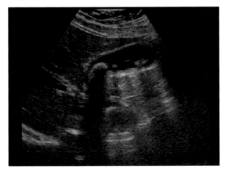

Ultrasound of cholelithiasis

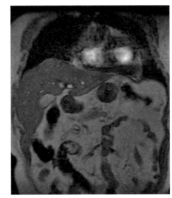

MRI: gallbladder

CHAPTER SEVEN   URINARY

7.0 Goals: Selecting the best studies to image the GU system

Objective questions:

7.1 When should I request a GU study?
7.2 What is an IVP and how is it performed?
7.3 How do I evaluate an IVP?
7.4 What are the IVP, CT, and ultrasound findings in obstructive uropathy?
7.5 What are the imaging findings in kidney cancer?
7.6 How can I be sure that a renal mass is truly cystic?
7.7 How can I locate the adrenal glands on CT and what are the common pathologies?
7.8 How is the prostate gland imaged?
7.9 How are the testicles imaged? What are the common pathologies?

7.1 When should I request a GU study?

Stone disease, infection, trauma, neoplasia, and vascular diseases are the most common maladies affecting the genitourinary system. Hematuria is a symptom that must be considered a sign of possible cancer anywhere from the kidney to the bladder. For this reason, cross-sectional imaging with CT, MRI, and/or ultrasound is important when screening for cancer.

Common reasons to request a genitourinary imaging study:

Kidney, ureter, or bladder calculus
Hematuria of unknown origin
Flank pain
Recurrent urinary tract infection
Suspected renal, ureteral, or bladder cancer
Scrotal mass
Suspected testicular torsion

7.2 What is an IVP and how is it performed?

An intravenous pyelogram (IVP), also known as an intravenous urogram, is an examination performed by the intravenous administration of iodinated contrast. Contrast is filtered by the kidneys, allowing for assessment of renal cortical function, filling of the renal collecting systems, the ureters, and the urinary bladder.

Urinary

Multiple films are obtained to demonstrate the sequential functioning of these structures. Recently, CT has supplanted IVP in many imaging centers because it is quick, accurate, and allows for more detailed assessment of renal anatomy. Cysts and tumors are more accurately evaluated with CT. Ultrasound is helpful for confirming a renal mass as a cyst and for detecting a dilated intrarenal collecting system (hydronephrosis).

TEACHING POINT

In many centers, CT has supplanted IVP for the assessment of stone disease and obstructive uropathy.

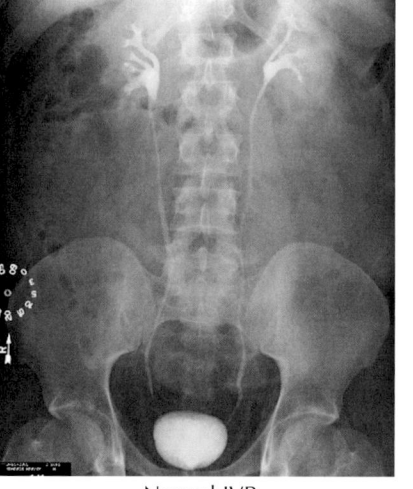

Normal IVP

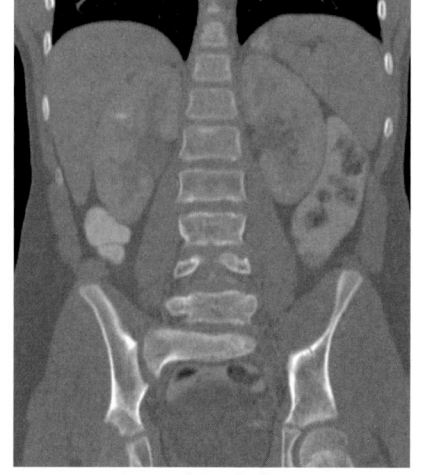

Coronal CT: kidneys

7.3 How do I evaluate an IVP?

The following steps can be used as a general guide for evaluating an IVP. An IVP is one of the few X-ray tests that allow us to determine the function of an organ. Most other imaging studies are simply static images that provide anatomic detail.

1. The scout films should be reviewed looking specifically for mineral (calcium) density overlying the kidneys or along the expected course of the ureters.
2. After contrast is given, radiographs are obtained at 1, 3, 5, and 10 minutes.
3. By 1 minute, the glomeruli and tubules begin to opacify (nephrographic phase).
4. By 5 minutes, the calyces and renal pelvis should be seen bilaterally (pyelographic phase). If there is an obstruction, a delay in the pyelographic phase on the affected side will be noted.
5. By 10 minutes, the ureters and bladder are visible. If there is obstruction, the ureter on the affected side may not yet be opacified or it may be seen to be dilated (ureterectasis).
6. If there is an obstruction, it may be necessary to obtain delayed radiographs up to several hours in an attempt to visualize the ureter and the site of obstruction.
7. The bladder should be distended by 10 minutes. Assess the bladder for filling defects that may reflect a stone or tumor.
8. Finally, the postvoid film is obtained to determine the ability of the patient to empty the bladder.

Urinary

7.4 What are the IVP, CT, and ultrasound signs of obstructive uropathy?

Any of these three imaging modalities may be used to detect obstruction of the urinary tract. Choose an IVP if you are interested in evaluation of renal function, CT if you suspect a kidney/ureteral calculus or renal tumor, and ultrasound if you wish to avoid radiation.

Summary of imaging findings in obstructive uropathy:

IVP:
1. Delay in the nephrographic and/or pyelographic phase.
2. Distention of the calyces, renal pelvis, and ureter to the level of the obstruction.

CT:
1. Contrast distention of the calyces and pelvis on the obstructed side.
2. Distention of the ureter to the site of obstruction.

Ultrasound:
1. Distention of the renal pelvis and calyces. The urine is anechoic (free of echoes) within the dilated collecting system.
2. The appearance of the pelvis and calyceal distention is likened to a bear paw.

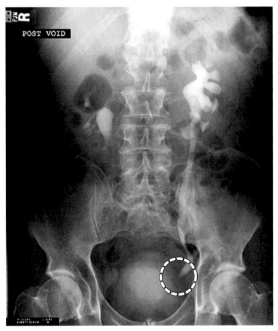

Left ureteral obstruction

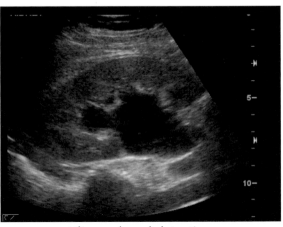

Ultrasound: renal obstruction

119

Urinary

7.5 What are the imaging findings in kidney cancer?

A renal mass will occasionally be visible on the abdominal plain film. When the plain film or the IVP is evaluated, the renal margins should be closely scrutinized. Kidney cancer most often presents with an abnormal contour bulge.

With CT, renal malignancy presents as a soft tissue mass that is solid and often lobulated. The lesion may be identical in density to the normal renal parenchyma on the noncontrasted images. With contrast, the kidney tumor becomes visible, often displaying areas of nonuniform enhancement. Renal neoplasms are extremely vascular. Rapid growth may outstrip the blood supply, resulting in central areas of low density, indicating tumor necrosis within the mass. The contour of the kidney is usually distorted and the collecting system is compressed and/or displaced. MRI will also demonstrate variations in signal intensity within a renal malignancy. CTA or MRA can be helpful to depict the relationship of the tumor to the renal artery or arteries (there is frequently more than one artery supplying the kidney). Imaging must also address the possibility of tumor invasion into the renal vein or inferior vena cava. Both contrast CT and MRI can detect this invasion, demonstrating a filling defect occupying the vessel lumen.

Ultrasound is excellent for distinguishing cyst from solid. All solid lesions are suspect for malignancy. Any complex cyst—that is, a cyst that has septa, wall thickening, or internal debris or contains a soft tissue mass—must be regarded as potentially malignant. If an ultrasound uncovers a solid renal mass or complex cyst, CT or MRI will then be indicated for further evaluation.

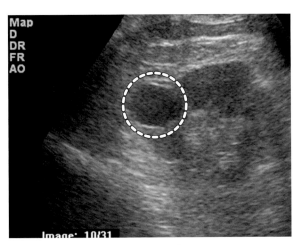

Ultrasound: renal cyst

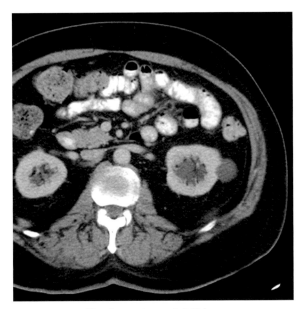

Simple renal cyst: left kidney

Urinary

7.6 How can I be sure that a renal mass is truly cystic?

It is important to confirm that a renal cystic lesion is simple. A simple cyst is always benign, but some cystic lesions are malignant. CT, ultrasound, or MRI can be used to confirm simple renal cyst.

A simple cyst on CT

1. Has no perceptible wall.
2. Has CT density measurements of 0.
3. Has no septa, mural nodules, or internal debris.
4. Is sharply circumscribed and round or oval in shape.

A simple cyst on MRI

1. Has no perceptible wall.
2. Is composed of water signal on all sequences (bright on T2, black on T1).
3. Has no septa, mural nodules, or internal debris.
4. Is sharply circumscribed and round or oval in shape.

A simple cyst on ultrasound

1. Is completely void of internal echoes.
2. Is round or oval in shape.
3. Displays increased through-transmission of sound.

7.7 How can I locate the adrenal glands on CT and what are the common pathologies?

The adrenal glands are located just superior and medial to the kidneys, usually on the 2–3 slices above the tops of the kidneys. These small structures can be hard to find in thin patients who do not have much intrabdominal fat. The adrenal glands are composed of two or three thin limbs that intersect at a small circular hilum. They most often have the shape of the letter Y or V. Adrenal adenomas are the most common adrenal pathology seen on CT. Adenomas are round or oval masses that are of slightly lower attenuation than the normal adrenal tissue because approximately 70% of them are composed of a partial lipoid matrix. Adrenal hyperplasia is also fairly common, presenting with diffuse thickening of the adrenal limbs. Primary adrenal carcinoma is relatively rare. These masses are usually larger than 2 cm and may have a necrotic center. More common is adrenal metastasis. In fact, adrenal metastasis in lung cancer is common enough that we always include the adrenal glands on all chest CT scans.

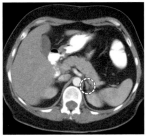

CT: normal adrenal gland

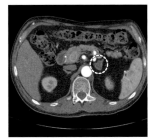

Left adrenal nodule

Urinary

7.8 How is the prostate gland imaged?

The prostate gland is well studied with ultrasound using a rectal probe. Well-defined zones of anatomy are easily demonstrated by ultrasound. Biopsy can be performed using this same specialized ultrasound probe.

MRI is also an excellent modality for the prostate gland. A specialized rectal coil is employed to provide excellent MR signal detail. MRI is especially useful for staging known prostate cancer.

Ultrasound is most often employed

As a screening test
To follow up an elevation of the prostate-specific antigen (PSA)
To study a palpable prostate nodule
To guide biopsy

7.9 How are the testicles imaged? What are the common pathologies?

Scrotal ultrasound is a quick and painless way to image the scrotal contents. Fluid accumulation (hydrocele) is easily identified. Doppler ultrasound is used to confirm arterial flow to the testes. Common pathologies that can be detected with scrotal ultrasound include hydrocele, vericocele, spermatocele, testicle torsion, epididymitis, and testicle tumors. Torsion of the testicle is an emergency that requires early detection to prevent infarction and irreversible testis damage.

8.0 Goals: Understanding how and when to image the GI tract

Objective questions:

8.1 What modalities are used in evaluating the GI system?
8.2 What is an esophagram and when should I order it?
8.3 What is an upper GI and how is it used?
8.4 How is the small intestine studied radiographically?
8.5 How is the colon imaged and how is barium enema used in practice?
8.6 What are the uses and limitations of barium studies?
8.7 What are the optimal examinations for specific evaluation of the gallbladder, liver, pancreas, and spleen?
8.8 What does esophageal cancer look like on an esophagram?
8.9 What does an ulcer look like on an upper GI?
8.10 What are the barium enema findings in colon cancer, diverticulitis, ulcerative colitis, and polyps?

Gastrointestinal

8.1 What modalities are used in evaluating the GI system?

Usually, the first imaging modality used to study the GI tract is a plain X-ray of the abdomen. Even when other GI examinations are planned, we frequently begin with plain films, or *scouts,* of the abdomen. The scout is used to assess the bowel gas pattern, to look for pathologic calcifications, and especially to determine whether the bowel has been adequately cleared of stool before a more specialized imaging test can be administered.

The barium esophagram is performed through the ingestion of opaque contrast. The contrast coats the esophageal mucosa and forms a temporary cast of the internal features of the esophagus.

An upper GI series uses the same technique as an esophagram, but the imaging is carried through to the duodenum. The patient is asked not to drink or eat after midnight the evening before the examination.

A barium enema is performed through a rectal tube. Contrast is administered retrograde through the colon to the cecum or the terminal ileum. Again, the temporary cast made by the contrast allows us to detect areas of constriction from cancer or inflammatory disease, areas of barium filling such as diverticulosis or ulcers, and areas of filling defects such as polyps.

CT is excellent for the solid visceral organs of the GI tract, the liver and pancreas. CT is not as good as barium studies for most bowel problems or as good as ultrasound for the gallbladder. CT is excellent for diagnosing appendicitis, diverticulitis, and pancreatitis.

The primary role of MRI is to provide additional information when the CT scan is equivocal. MRI is used to image inflammatory bowel disease such as Crohn's disease. It can help clarify disease processes in the solid visceral organs.

There are two main reasons why the gallbladder is best imaged with ultrasound. First, the gallbladder is a fluid-filled structure, and evaluating fluid collections is the forte of ultrasound. Second, the gallbladder, being located adjacent to a solid, easily recognized structure like the liver, is easy to find sonographically. In addition, the extrahepatic and intrahepatic bile ducts are nicely imaged with ultrasound.

Gastrointestinal

8.2 What is an esophagram and when should I order it?

An esophagram, also called a *barium swallow,* is performed by having the patient swallow barium, which is an inert, nonabsorbable mineral that creates an easily identifiable opacity on X-rays. (The patient must be able to drink fluids safely.) The column of contrast is followed through its course in the esophagus and X-ray pictures are obtained in multiple projections in all areas of the esophagus. When mixed with water, barium forms a chalky liquid that can distend the hollow structures of the gastrointestinal tract and coat its mucosa. All barium studies are based on the principle of forming a cast of the hollow organ. The barium suspension insinuates itself into the mucosal folds. If a mass is present, it can displace the barium, resulting in a filling defect. In the opposite way, an ulcer crater is a hole that is filled up with barium and presents on the X-ray as a projection of barium into the nonopacified bowel wall.

Reasons to order an esophagram:

   Dysphagia (difficulty swallowing)
   Odynophagia (painful swallowing)
   Foreign body sensation, food or other foreign body
   Chest pain suspected to be related to gastroesophageal reflux disease (GERD)
   Esophageal cancer
   Zenker's diverticulum
   Hiatal hernia
   Barrett's esophagus

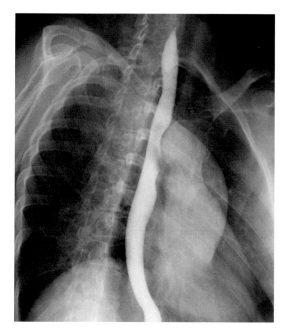

Normal esophagram (oblique view)

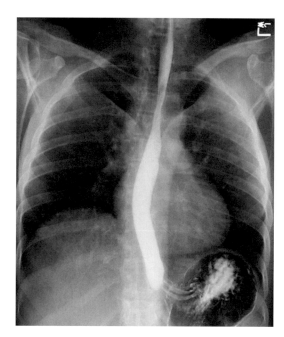

Normal esophagram (AP view)

8.3 What is an upper GI and when is it used?

In an upper GI, the patient swallows barium and the radiologist performs real-time X-rays (fluoroscopy). Barium can be followed from the mouth to the duodenum. Static X-ray images are obtained documenting the course, caliber, and distention of the esophagus, stomach, and duodenum. *Single contrast* indicates that only the barium suspension is used to form a cast of these hollow organs. *Double contrast* indicates the use of both barium and air, which is introduced into the stomach by carbon dioxide-releasing crystals. The air allows the mucosa to be coated by a thin layer of barium, providing a much more sensitive and accurate means to detect mucosal disease such as polyps and ulceration. There is usually no need to specify air-contrast upper GI on your orders, since most radiologists use it unless the patient is unable to tolerate it because of age or other factors.

Reasons to order an upper GI:

Abdominal pain
Gastric or duodenal ulcer
Bezoar
Mass pathology
Gastric obstruction

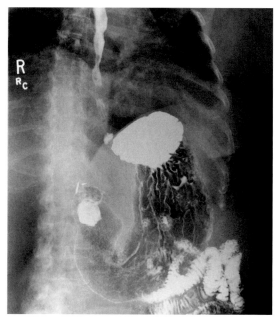

Normal air contrast—upper GI

8.4 How is the small intestine studied radiographically?

There are two common ways to study the small intestine without CT. The most common method is a *small bowel follow-through* (SBFT), which is performed just as it sounds. A barium suspension is given by mouth and serial abdominal radiographs are obtained as the contrast traverses the small intestine. The study is concluded when the barium reaches the colon and—because of the propensity for Crohn's disease to affect the distal small bowel—specific spot radiographs are obtained to document the terminal ileum and the ileocecal valve. The second method, *enteroclysis,* is more time-consuming but also more accurate. A long tube is inserted through the nose or mouth and positioned at the junction of the duodenum and jejunum as marked by the upper sweep of the fourth arm of the duodenum. A bolus of thick contrast is injected through the tube, followed by a methyl cellulose solution (not visible on X-rays). This solution pushes the contrast forward, coats the small intestinal mucosa, and distends the bowel for accurate assessment of the mucosa. Enteroclysis is reserved for difficult cases, small bowel tumors, polyps, or conditions where fine mucosal detail would be helpful. Consider ordering a small bowel study for

Chronic diarrhea
Gluten sensitivity (nontropical sprue)
Small bowel lymphoma or other suspected malignancy
Weight loss of unknown cause
Steatorrhea (fatty stool)
Inflammatory bowel disease

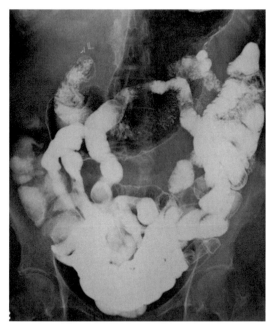

Normal small bowel follow-through

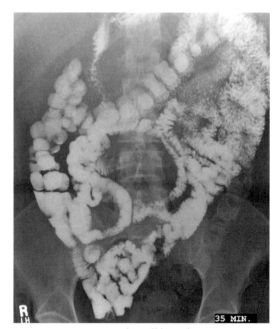

Normal small bowel

Gastrointestinal

8.5 How is the colon imaged and how is barium enema used in practice?

Colonoscopy has replaced barium enema, with a few exceptions, because it is a little more sensitive for the detection of polyps and because biopsy can be performed at the time of colonoscopy. Barium enema is used if the endoscope cannot be advanced all the way to the cecum. Water-soluble contrast is used if obstruction is suspected and rapid diagnosis is required. Barium enema can be an initial screening test in those few patients who refuse colonoscopy. A single-contrast barium enema is performed by gravity drainage of a barium-filled enema bag into the colon. The contrast is followed by fluoroscopy (real time X-ray imaging) to the cecum. Multiple X-ray views are taken. Because polyps are better seen with double contrast, most barium enemas are completed using a combination of thick barium (to coat the mucosa) and air (to distend the colon).

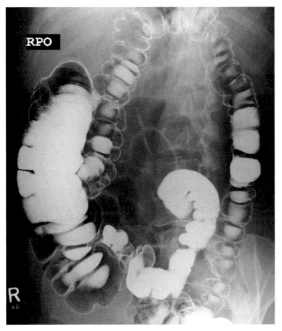

Normal air contrast: barium enema

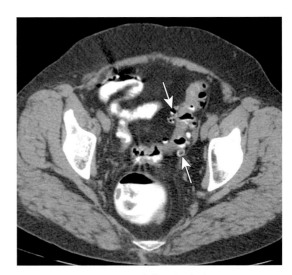

CT: sigmoid diverticulosis

Gastrointestinal

8.6 What are the uses and limitations of barium studies?

The barium studies discussed above—esophagram, upper GI, small bowel follow-through, and barium enema—are often performed for screening purposes or on occasion to confirm or reevaluate a finding seen during endoscopy. Because the radiologist watches the barium column in real time with fluoroscopy, physiologic information such as peristalsis can be obtained.

Barium examinations are excellent for evaluating the caliber of hollow viscera. Areas of narrowing can be evaluated for their length and contour. Strictures with irregular margins raise concern for cancer. Inflammatory strictures can be identified anywhere from the esophagus to the rectum.

Filling defects such as polyps or masses create an area of contour abnormality. However, while we can predict whether a stricture, polyp, or mass appears to be benign or malignant, only biopsy can provide a definitive answer. Endoscopy has the advantage of the option for biopsy or treatment. Barium studies are diagnostic only. In addition, endoscopy is at least as accurate as barium examinations, and most physicians believe that it is more accurate.

8.7 What are the optimal examinations for specific evaluation of the gallbladder, liver, pancreas, and spleen?

Once you have decided to image a specific organ, the next important consideration is how best to study it. The gallbladder, being a fluid-filled structure, is best imaged with ultrasound. When you request a gallbladder ultrasound, you will also get information about the liver, bile ducts, right kidney, and pancreas. There are few if any contraindications to gallbladder ultrasound.

Gallbladder ultrasound should be performed prior to a HIDA scan, especially when a gallbladder ejection fraction is requested. The HIDA scan is a nuclear imaging study that gives information about the patency of the cystic duct and common bile duct. The HIDA scan is especially useful for the diagnosis of acute cholecystitis (edema results in occlusion of the cystic duct and therefore no tracer will be seen in the gallbladder) and chronic cholecystitis (delayed visualization of the gallbladder). The nuclear HIDA scan provides excellent physiologic information but limited anatomic detail. Once the radio tracer has accumulated in the gallbladder, an intravenous injection of a gallbladder-stimulating compound allows the technologist to calculate the gallbladder ejection fraction. This physiologic information is helpful to determine the functional status (contractility) of the gallbladder.

The liver, pancreas, and spleen are best imaged with CT. Although ultrasound can provide excellent information, overlying gas often obscures portions of these organs. If CT is equivocal, MRI is the best imaging study to clarify a finding or to help refine the differential diagnosis.

Gastrointestinal

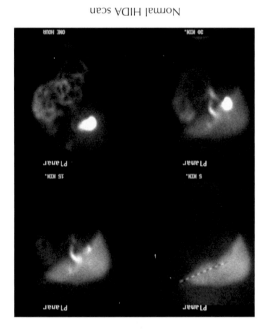

Normal gallbladder ultrasound

Normal HIDA scan

8.8 What does esophageal cancer look like on an esophagram?

The most common presentation of esophageal cancer is an asymmetric stricture of the lower esophagus. The barium cast of the esophageal lumen is narrow and irregular. There are often small ulcerations where barium collects, as well as areas of irregular filling defects. The proximal portion of the esophagus may be dilated from the obstruction. Varicoid carcinoma can occur in the stomach or the esophagus, presenting as wormlike filling defects that may be confused with varices. Early esophageal cancer can be as subtle as segmental mucosal roughening or irregularity. Inflammatory esophageal strictures present with smooth, symmetrical luminal narrowing. Whether a stricture is thought to be benign or malignant from an imaging standpoint, endoscopy with mucosal biopsy is always indicated.

8.9 What does an ulcer look like on an upper GI?

An ulcer is a hole in the mucosa that collects barium contrast. The rim of the ulcer is often edematous, creating a smooth, collar-like surrounding filling defect. An ulcer in the stomach should always raise concern for carcinoma. Gastric carcinoma often presents with ulceration. The filling defect of the gastric mass may be more subtle than the ulcer itself. An ulcer in the duodenum is most often inflammatory (peptic ulcer disease). The adjacent mucosa may be edematous and the mucosal folds thickened. Punctate ulcerations are pinpoint contrast collections. Seen head on, ulcers present like targets: a central opaque barium-containing ulcer crater and a surrounding low-density rim or collar. Seen in profile, ulcers are seen as projections of barium into the mucosa.

8.10 What are the barium enema findings in colon cancer, diverticulitis, ulcerative colitis, and polyps?

The typical colon cancer encircles the lumen of the colon, producing the aptly named finding of an "apple core" lesion. This localized luminal constriction displays irregular margins like tooth marks on an apple core. It is also sometimes called a "napkin ring" because of the abrupt change in the caliber of the bowel lumen. When colon cancer presents earlier, there may be an irregular elevation of the mucosa. In the rectum, the appearance of raised nodular mucosa when seen in profile is referred to as a "carpet lesion." In any case, the normally smooth contour of barium and air adjacent to the smooth colon mucosa is irregular and microlobulated.

A diverticulum is an out-pouching of the colon wall. A noninflamed diverticulum appears as a smoothly margined sac-like structure with a narrow waist and broad balloon-like body. Diverticula may occur anywhere from the esophagus to the rectum, but they are most common by far in the sigmoid colon. When inflamed, the smooth sac is replaced by a jagged triangular or thorn-shaped barium collection. As the mucosal inflammation continues, this sawtooth pattern is often accompanied by constriction of the colon lumen.

Ulcerative colitis is a diffuse inflammatory process involving bowel mucosa. Early in the process, the ulcerations are tiny, producing granular defects in the mucosa. As the ulcers deepen, they can resemble small diverticula, or so-called collar-button ulcers. Diffuse mucosal involvement is present, while in the skip lesions of Crohn's disease it is not. In addition, the rectum is almost always affected by ulcerative colitis and less commonly in Crohn's disease. Care must be taken when ordering a barium enema in acute ulcerative colitis, as the enema may precipitate toxic megacolon, a state of severe colitis with marked colon distention, placing the colon at risk for perforation and/or ischemia. Late-stage ulcerative colitis results in a smooth, featureless colon mucosa secondary to chronic inflammation. This appearance on barium enema has been referred to as a "pipestem" colon.

Polyps in the GI tract are small filling defects. They may appear as small broad-based bumps on the mucosa, sessile polyps, or on a stalk as pedunculated polyps. Small polyps less than 5 mm in size are easily overlooked on a barium enema. These are often hyperplastic polyps without malignant potential. Adenomatous polyps are usually larger than 5 mm and do carry a risk of harboring adenocarcinoma.

CHAPTER NINE   MUSCULOSKELETAL

9.0 Goals: Understanding the indications and modalities used for imaging the musculoskeletal system and basic interpretation skills

Objective questions:

9.1 What modalities are used to evaluate bones and joints?
9.2 How do I find a fracture on an X-ray?
9.3 How can I best describe fractures?
9.4 What is the Salter-Harris classification of growth plate fractures?
9.5 What is dislocation and how can I recognize and describe it?
9.6 What does arthritis look like on an X-ray?
9.7 How is osteomyelitis diagnosed?
9.8 How are bone tumors classified and described?
9.9 When is CT better than plain film X-rays?
9.10 When is CT better than MRI?
9.11 When should I order an MRI?

9.1 What modalities are used to evaluate bones and joints?

X-ray modalities (plain film and CT) are excellent for studying the detail of cortical and trabecular bone. Soft issues, including cartilage, ligaments, tendons, muscles, and bone marrow, are usually best imaged with MRI. Nuclear imaging gives us less anatomic information but more physiologic data. A bone scan is performed by injecting a material that is readily taken up by actively growing bone. This material has been tagged with a radioactive pharmaceutical that decays and produces a gamma ray, which in turn can be imaged by a gamma camera. Actively growing bone can be found in healing fractures, in tumors, and around infections. These areas are said to be "hot" on a bone scan because there will be a greater concentration of the radiopharmaceutical.

Musculoskeletal

Summary of bone and joint imaging modalities:

> Plain film radiographs
> CT
> MRI
> Nuclear bone scanning

9.2 How do I find a fracture on an X-ray?

I suggest a three-step process in the evaluation of bones and soft tissues for the signs of fracture. The first, and perhaps the most sensitive, is the assessment of the soft tissues for swelling or signs of joint effusion, mainly displacement of intra-articular fat pads. The last two involve the careful scrutiny of cortical continuity and contour abnormalities.

Three-step process to find a fracture on X-ray:

> Start with soft tissues, looking for swelling or fat pad displacement.
> Examine the cortex along the entire length of the bone.
> Look for cortical irregularity, buckling, or evidence of impaction.

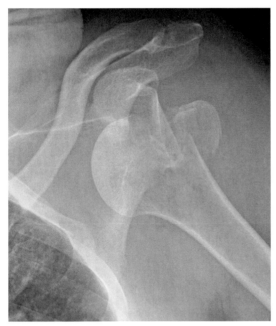

Fracture-dislocation—right humeral head

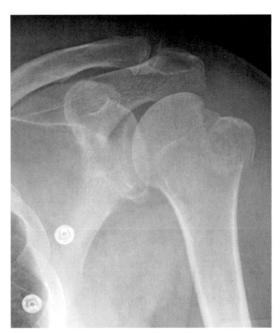

Reduction films

Musculoskeletal

9.3 How can I best describe fractures?

The primary goal of fracture description is to paint an accurate verbal picture of the injury. Once you have identified the fracture line, determine whether it extends completely through the bone (complete versus incomplete). Next, evaluate the course of the fracture line: transverse, oblique, longitudinal, or spiral. Determine if there is displacement or angulation of the distal fracture fragment. The term *comminuted* applies if there are more than two pieces of bone or more than one fracture line. Look closely at the articular surfaces nearest the fracture. If the fracture line extends into a joint, it is very important to communicate this finding so that all efforts can be made to restore alignment along the articular surface. Finally, if bone is exposed to air, either because of associated laceration or because the fragment protrudes through the skin, this is an open fracture at risk for infection.

Fracture description checklist of long bone fracture descriptors:

Direction of the fracture line: transverse, oblique, longitudinal, spiral
Displacement
Angulation
Comminution
Articular involvement
Open or closed

Summary of fracture recognition and description

1. Check the name, date, and orientation of the part being examined.
2. Get a global impression of the study, noting alignment, bone density, and any gross deformity.
3. Carefully examine the soft tissues for swelling, foreign body, or soft tissue air.
4. Look for displacement of fat pads around all joints. A positive posterior fat pad in the elbow is always regarded as a fracture even if the fracture itself is not visible.
5. Follow the dense white cortex of bone along each and every surface of visible bone and on all three projections (AP, lateral, and oblique).
6. Examine articular relationships for subluxation or dislocation of a joint.

Common Types of Fractures

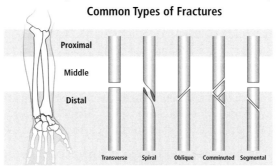

Fracture patterns

Musculoskeletal

9.4 What is the Salter-Harris classification of growth plate fractures?

Salter and Harris were prominent Canadian surgeons who recognized, described, and classified specific patterns of growth plate injury in children (1963). There are nine categories of injury, but only five occur frequently enough to be in general use for most practitioners. Detecting and classifying these injuries is important to allow for the prediction of potential functional disability resulting from the growth plate damage. *Type I* is separation of the epiphysis from the metaphysis. The fracture line travels across the growth plate and results in a gap between the epiphysis and the metaphysis. This finding can be very subtle and may require a comparison view of the opposite limb to be recognized. Functional disability is rare. *Type II* is the most common Salter-Harris injury. The fracture line extends partially through the growth plate and then travels obliquely through the metaphysis. Functional disability is uncommon. A *type III* fracture extends longitudinally through the epiphysis to the growth plate. Because the fracture extends to the articular surface, the possibility of future disability is greater than with types I and II. *Type IV* is a fracture that extends longitudinally through the epiphysis and also obliquely through the metaphysis. This injury has components of both types II and III and may result in disability due to joint involvement. *Type V* is a compression injury of the growth plate. This too is a subtle injury that is recognized by narrowing of the growth plate when compared to other growth plates. This crush injury may result in growth disturbance because of premature closure of the growth plate.

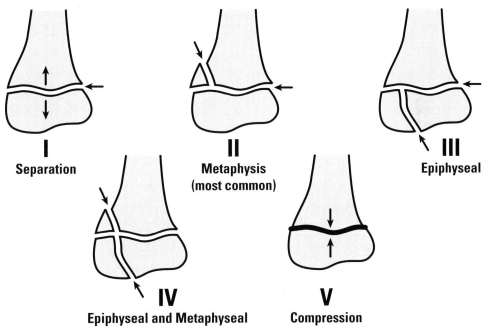

I

Separation

II

Metaphysis
(most common)

III

Epiphyseal

IV

Epiphyseal and Metaphyseal

V

Compression

Salter-Harris classification

Musculoskeletal

9.5 What is dislocation and how can I recognize and describe it?

Dislocation is complete displacement of a bone from its articulation (joint). An anterior or subcoracoid dislocation of the humerus is most common in the shoulder. A posterior dislocation of the radius and/or ulna is most common in the elbow. A posterior dislocation is also the most common way the femoral head is dislocated in the hip. The patella tends to dislocate in a lateral direction. The talus most often dislocates laterally in the ankle.

Dislocation is recognized when anatomic alignment of the joint is lost. In the shoulder, on the AP view, the dislocated humerus is seen to lie inferior to the coracoid process of the scapula rather than its usual position below the acromion. A scapular "Y" or axillary view should be obtained to help you determine that the humeral head is anteriorly displaced. Posterior dislocation of the shoulder is more difficult to detect, especially on the AP view. It tends to occur because of an intense muscular contraction of back muscles, such as during a grand mal seizure or electric shock. Therefore, the AP view alone is not sufficient: the standard views of the shoulder include an AP in internal rotation, an AP with external rotation, and a scapular "Y" projection.

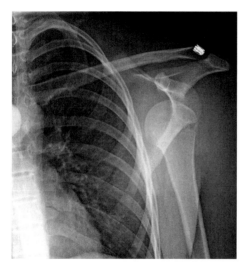

Anterior subcoracoid shoulder dislocation

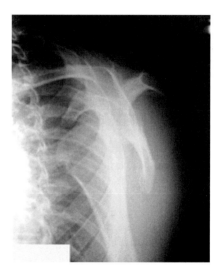

Scapular "Y" view of anterior dislocation

Musculoskeletal

9.6 What does arthritis look like on an X-ray?

Arthritis can be divided into two categories: *degenerative* (or *osteoarthritis*) and *inflammatory*. In osteoarthritis, the joint space narrows and the bone reacts to the increased pressure by becoming dense (sclerosis) and by forming para-articular new bone (osteophytes). Osteoarthritis can affect any joint, but it is common in the hips and knees and the facet joints of the spine. It favors the distal interphalangeal joints of the hand.

Inflammatory arthritis includes rheumatoid arthritis, gout, pseudogout, psoriatic arthritis, and septic arthritis. In these conditions, there is usually some degree of joint destruction and osseous erosion. Increased blood flow (hyperemia) results in diminished bone density adjacent to the joint (juxta-articular osteopenia). Inflammatory synovium erodes bone at the margins of the joint where cartilage does not cover the bone (bare areas). The joint space narrows, ligaments become lax, and, late in the disease, characteristic subluxations occur. In rheumatoid arthritis, the proximal phylangeal articulations of the hand are more commonly involved than the distal joints.

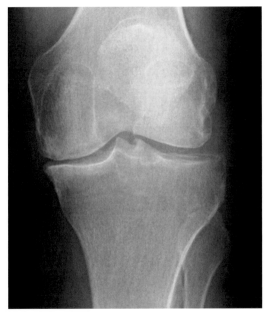

Degenerative joint disease, left knee

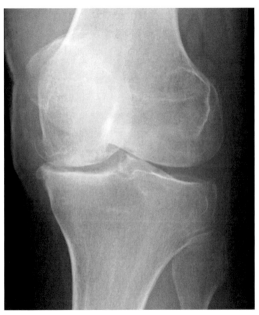

Degenerative osteophytes—medial femur and tibia

Musculoskeletal

9.7 How is osteomyelitis diagnosed?

Plain X-rays are usually the first step in imaging. Para-articular soft tissue swelling and joint effusion present as hazy fluid accumulation around a joint that may displace normal fat pads. The periosteum may thicken or may be elevated away from the cortex. The osseous structure loses density (osteopenia). Bone destruction, however, is the only primary sign of osteomyelitis. When bone begins to vanish, the infection has usually been present for weeks. A bone scan or MRI is much more sensitive than a plain film for the detection of early osteomyelitis. With bone scanning, a three-phase technique is used. Technetium 99m is tagged to MDP (methyldiphosphonate) and injected intravenously. A flow study is the first phase. It will demonstrate increased vascular flow to the area of infection. Early (immediately after the injection) and delayed (three to six hours after the injection) imaging will demonstrate progressive, intense uptake of the MDP into the area of infection as the bone struggles to rebuild from the destructive process. MRI demonstrates increased fluid in and around the area of osteomyelitis. The bone marrow will become less intense on T1 (fluid) and more intense on T2. When gadolinium contrast is administered, there is enhancement of the inflammatory tissues.

9.8 How are bone tumors classified and described?

Bone tumors are classified in several ways. First, the tumor may be *benign* or *malignant*. If the tumor is malignant, the aggressiveness of disease can be predicted with plain film, CT, and MRI findings. Malignant tumors are further classified as *primary* and *metastatic*. It is extremely important to consider the age of the patient. Bone tumors occur predictably within certain age ranges, and they characteristically occur in specific areas. Diagnosing a bone tumor is like picking real estate. The three most important factors are location, location, and location.

Certain primary tumors tend to spread to bone, such as breast and prostate cancer. Metastatic lesions are classified as *lytic* (causing destruction) or *blastic* (associated with dense metastatic tissue elements).

There are three key descriptors of bone tumors. In order of least aggressive to most aggressive, they are *geographic, moth-eaten,* and *permeative*. A geographic tumor is well-defined and has a sharp zone of transition and sclerotic borders (an example is a fibroxanthoma). A moth-eaten tumor is more aggressive. The zone of transition between the tumor and normal bone is less clear and there are no sclerotic margins (an example is multiple myeloma). A permeative tumor is the most aggressive. There is no visible wall, the transition from tumor to normal bone is obscure, and the periosteum is often pushed to become at right angles to the bone (an example is osteosarcoma).

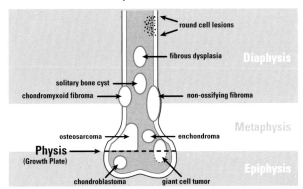

Distribution of bone tumors

Musculoskeletal

9.9 When is CT better than plain film X-rays?

CT has the advantage of computer-generated three-dimensional reconstruction. Thin-section CT gives great anatomic detail of cortical and medullary bone without overlapping tissue shadows. The following fractures are best characterized using CT:

> Tibial plateau fracture, especially with coronal reconstruction, to look for depression or displacement of a fracture fragment
> Acetabular fracture
> Calcaneal fracture
> Facial bone or orbital fracture
> Talar fracture
> Sternal fracture, especially with coronal reconstruction

9.10 When is CT better than MRI?

CT is better than MRI when we are looking at the relationships between cortical bone and joint surfaces in the acetabulum and tibial plateau or when there may be multiple complex fracture lines. The key word is *cortical* bone. The cortex is white and easy to see on CT and is devoid of signal with MRI.

9.11 When should I request an MRI?

When you think of soft tissue imaging, think MRI. Soft tissue includes not only muscle, tendon, ligament, and cartilage, but also bone marrow. Fluid collections are easy to see on an MRI. Fluid presents with bright white signal on T2-weighted images.

Suspected muscle, tendon, cartilage, or ligament tears
Bone marrow disorders
Suspected stress or radiographically occult fracture
Soft tissue or bone tumors
Ischemic necrosis

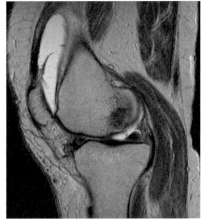

MRI suprapatellar effusion

Musculoskeletal

9.12 When is a bone scan indicated?

Bone scanning is physiologic imaging of living bone. Bone scans are indicated for

> Stress fracture
> Radiographically occult fracture
> Osteomyelitis
> Osseous metastatic disease (blastic type)
> Prosthesis loosening

9.13 Postural evaluation: what is the procedure to evaluate for leg-length discrepancy?

A postural study is used to estimate leg length, sacral base tilting, and lumbosacral angle. An AP film of the pelvis is obtained with the patient standing. A plumb line (a thin chain with a weight on the end) is pinned to the patient's gown for reference, and the difference in heights between the two lines is measured drawing a perpendicular line from the plumb line to the superior margin of each femoral head. If the femoral heads are on the same plane, there is no leg-length discrepancy.

To evaluate the sacral base plane, on the same AP film of the pelvis a line is drawn connecting dots at the lowest point of the sacral sulcus on the left and right. If this line is perpendicular to the plumb line, there is no sacral base tilt (normal).

The weightbearing line is constructed on a lateral view of the lumbar spine. With normal alignment, a line drawn parallel to the plumb line should fall from the midbody of L3 to the anterior third of the sacral base.

9.14 What is a scanogram?

A scanogram is an X-ray examination performed in the AP projection with a specialized ruler included in the radiograph. It is the most accurate X-ray method to measure leg length. The femurs are measured from the superior margin of the femoral head to the inferior margin of the medial femoral condyle. The tibiae are measured from the medial tibial plateau to the articular margin of the distal tibia.

Musculoskeletal

9.15 How do I examine the cervical spine?

There are five basic views of the cervical spine: lateral, AP, left oblique, right oblique, and open-mouth odontoid. The lateral view is the most important because it contains information about vertebral alignment, integrity of the cortex, heights of the vertebral bodies, and presence of precervical soft tissue swelling. The steps to follow in evaluating the cervical spine X-ray are as follows:

1. Count the segments. You should see as far inferiorly as T1 and always C7.
2. Examine alignment (anteriorly and posteriorly). Alignment is assessed by closely examining the three arcs of the cervical spine. See figure.
3. Examine the precervical soft tissues (normal up to 6 mm at C2 and 22 mm at C6).
4. Follow the cortex of each vertebral segment.
5. Compare disk spaces at each level.
6. Identify the odontoid process on lateral and open-mouth views
7. Check for alignment of the lateral masses of C1 and C2 on the open-mouth odontoid view.
8. Check for midline position of the spinous processes on the AP view.

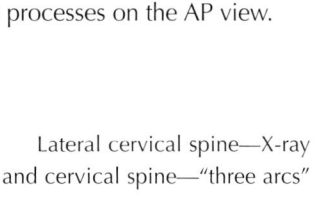

MEMORY JOGGER

"6 at 2 and 22 at 6," referring to the upper normal soft tissue measurement between the cervical spine and the airway at C2 and at C6.

Lateral cervical spine—X-ray and cervical spine—"three arcs"

9.16 How do I examine the thoracic spine?

AP and lateral views are standard in thoracic spine radiography.

1. On the AP view, count the number of thoracic segments and corresponding ribs.
2. On the AP view, check each pedicle. The pedicles are seen as oval structures on either side of the vertebral bodies. Metastatic disease favors the pedicles.
3. On the AP view, look at the soft tissues on each side of the thoracic spine for evidence of paraspinal mass pathology.
4. On the lateral, evaluate thoracic vertebral body heights and disk spaces.
5. Note the thoracic kyphosis—is it exaggerated?
6. Check the integrity of the cortex throughout the spine.

Musculoskeletal

9.17 How do I examine the lumbar spine?

There are five projections of the lumbar spine: AP, lateral, spot lateral at L5-S1, right oblique, and left oblique. The oblique views are helpful for visualization of the pars interarticularis (the part between the superior and inferior articulating facets). On the oblique view, the "Scottie dog" can be seen, named for the shape created by the articular facets, the pedicle, and the pars interarticularis (the neck of the Scottie dog). When the pacs interarticularis is fractured or congenitally absent, this is called a *pars defect* or *spondylolysis.* Bilateral spondylolysis can result in forward slipping of the upper vertebral body relative to the lower one. This slipping is called *spondylolesthesis* and is graded from I to IV.

Steps in evaluating the lumbar spine:

1. On the AP view, check vertebral alignment, pedicles, and transverse processes.
2. On the oblique views, check for spondylolysis and facet alignment.
3. On the lateral view, evaluate vertebral body heights and disk spaces.
4. Note the lumbar lordosis: is it flattened or exaggerated?
5. The spot lateral view at L5-S1 is done to give an accurate assessment of the disk space. The two most common areas for disk disease in the lumbar spine are L4–5 and L5-S1.

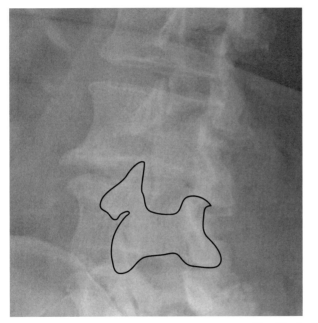
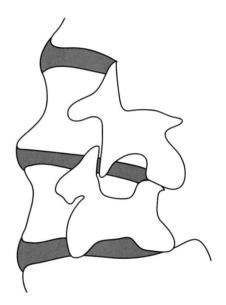

"Scottie dog"

Musculoskeletal

9.18 What is DEXA and how does it measure bone density?

Dual X-ray absorptometry is the method used to pass a known quantity of X-rays through the bones of the lumbar spine and hip. A computer compensates for the patient's body type and weight and then calculates the bones' ability to block the X-rays. The denser the bone, the more the X-rays will be blocked. Density measurements are calculated within each of the lower four vertebral bodies and within five areas of the hip. Bone mass density scoring relates the findings to the patient's score compared to a normal healthy female of any age (the T score) and also to female patients of the same age (the Z score).

Normal	T = –1.4 or higher
Osteopenia	T = –1.5 to –2.49
Osteoporosis	T = –2.5 or lower

10.0 Goals: Understanding how to image the head and neck

Objective questions:

10.1   What anatomy is visible of paranasal sinus radiography?
10.2   When should CT be ordered in the head and neck?
10.3   When is ultrasound helpful in the head and neck?
10.4   Is MRI useful in the head and neck?
10.5   What are the general types of facial bone injury and how are they imaged?
10.6   What is a blowout fracture of the orbit?
10.7   What is a tripod fracture?
10.8   What imaging tests are used to evaluate thyroid and parathyroid disease?

Head and Neck

10.1 What anatomy is visible on paranasal sinus radiography?

Plain X-rays of the paranasal sinuses allow us to assess the maxillary, ethmoid, frontal, and sphenoid sinuses. The nasal bones are best imaged in the lateral projection, and the nasal septum alignment is best seen on frontal radiographs. The pathologic findings seen on plain films of the face and sinuses relate primarily to facial bone fracture and soft tissue or fluid densities in the paranasal sinuses. Masses require cross-sectional imaging with CT, ultrasound, or MRI.

The best way for a student to learn head-and-neck imaging anatomy is to practice labeling structures. This can be accomplished on the Internet, where there are many excellent source images. When on the radiology service, ask for copies of imaging studies (patients' names removed) to practice labeling normal anatomy. Specialized wax pencils are available with which to do this.

10.2 When should CT be ordered in the head and neck?

CT is excellent for evaluation of the paranasal sinuses. Reserve CT for cases that do not respond to conventional therapy or for recurrent sinusitis. CT can accurately distinguish between chronic and acute sinusitis, demonstrate obstruction or patency of sinus ostia, and demonstrate bone destruction, turbinate size, and septum position. Sinus polyps, mucous retention cysts, and other tumors are well demonstrated. CT is also excellent for assessment of the salivary glands, neck masses, and laryngeal cancer as well as other cancers of the mouth, tongue, or pharynx.

CT is often used to evaluate facial bone fractures. The benefits include the ability to obtain three-dimensional computer reconstructions that permit surgeons to plan restorative therapy after facial injuries. In particular, orbital blowout fractures may not be clearly defined with plain films. CT can be performed in the axial plane, or, if the patient can tolerate neck extension or flexion, direct coronal imaging can be done.

10.3 When is ultrasound helpful in the head and neck?

Ultrasound is very accurate in the evaluation of the thyroid gland. The size of the gland, including volume measurements, can be accurately measured. Thyroid nodules can be quantified and measured, and distinction can be made between solid and cyst. Ultrasound is preferred for image-guided biopsy. As a general rule, solid, solitary nodules are more suspicious for malignancy than multiple nodules or cysts. Often, in a multinodular gland, the largest nodule(s) should undergo biopsy. It is not possible to distinguish a benign from a malignant nodule on the basis of ultrasound or any other imaging modality.

The parathyroid glands are often difficult to image with any modality. Ultrasound has the advantage of no radiation and good spatial resolution. The most common reason to image the parathyroid glands is elevation of serum calcium. Calcium can be elevated in parathyroid hyperplasia or parathyroid adenoma. Remember that calcium is also elevated in malignancies including lung cancer.

Ultrasound is also excellent in evaluation of the carotid arteries. This is most often requested if a bruit is heard or if there are signs or symptoms of transient ischemic attack or stroke. Magnetic resonance angiography and computed tomography angiography are fast becoming excellent ways to measure carotid stenosis.

Head and Neck

10.4 Is MRI useful in the head and neck?

The advantages of MRI in the head and neck are its lack of radiation and its multiplanar capability. With the patient in the supine position, images can be obtained in any plane. MRI is excellent in the evaluation of salivary glands and neck masses.

10.5 What are the general types of facial bone injury and how are they imaged?

Blunt and penetrating trauma can cause facial injury. As with all skeletal injuries, soft tissue findings are often very helpful clues to the site and the severity of the injury.

Most common facial bone fractures:

- Nasal bones
- Maxillary sinus
- Orbital floor
- Orbital wall
- Zygomatic arch

Classification of facial bone injuries:

- Tripod (zygomaticomaxillary complex) fracture
- LeFort fractures types I, II, and III
- Nasal bone fracture

Anterior maxillary spine fracture
Orbital blowout injuries
Smash fractures

Depending upon the severity of the injury and the clinical suspicion of intracranial hemorrhage, a decision must be made about using plain films (less severe trauma) or computed tomography (severe trauma). Without question, CT is more sensitive for the detection and more accurate for the characterization of facial fractures. Intracranial bleeding cannot be identified using plain films. Therefore, any trauma that raises concern for facial fracture with intracranial injury should be studied with CT. Whether the trauma is blunt or penetrating, plain film findings that alert the clinician to underlying fracture include malar soft tissue swelling, air-fluid leveling in the maxillary sinus, and air in the orbital cavity.

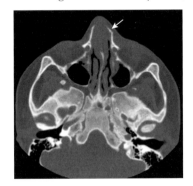

CT: nasal bone fracture

10.6 What is a blowout fracture of the orbit?

The orbit is a cone-shaped container housing the globe, the optic nerve, the extraocular muscles, and an abundant cushion of fat. When the orbit is struck by a blunt object such as a baseball, the pressure within the orbit rises abruptly, often causing fracture of the thinnest wall of the orbit: the medial wall or lamina papyrecea (paper-thin layer) and/or the orbital floor. In either case, the injury is called a *blowout fracture* and the orbital contents can herniate into the ethmoid sinus (medial wall blowout) or the maxillary sinus (orbital floor blowout). When the orbital floor is fractured, blood and herniated tissue bulge into the superior aspect of the maxillary sinus, producing a "hammock sign." This may entrap the inferior rectus muscle, causing double vision (diploplia). A blowout fracture can also allow air from the sinus to enter the orbit, resulting in the X-ray finding of orbital emphysema.

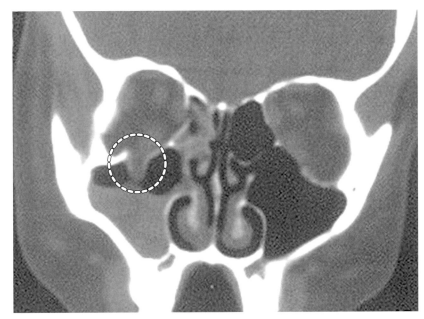

Orbital blowout fracture

Head and Neck

10.7 What is a tripod fracture?

The malar bone, also called the zygoma or cheek bone, is like a curved tabletop supported by three legs. The three legs are the frontal process of the zygoma, the zygomatic arch, and the lateral wall of the maxillary sinus. A direct blow to the malar bone can result in fracture of all three legs (tripod fracture). A tripod fracture is a common type of facial bone injury.

Three components of the tripod fracture:

Fracture of the zygomatic arch
Separation of the frontozygomatic suture
Fracture of the lateral maxillary sinus wall

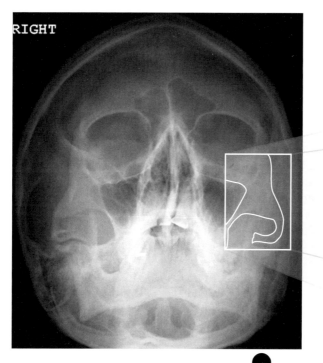

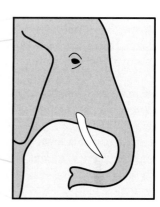

Malar bone
Elephant's trunk = zygomatic arch

10.8 What imaging tests are used to evaluate thyroid and parathyroid disease?

The two most common tests for studying the thyroid gland are a thyroid scan and ultrasound. A thyroid scan is a nuclear medicine test in which the patient is given an oral dose of radioactive iodine. The radioactive materials that may be used are techetium 99-m, iodine-123, and iodine-131. The radioactive iodine is taken up by the thyroid gland, and imaging is performed by a specialized gamma camera that measures the intensity of radiation coming from the gland. The size of the gland and the uniformity of the tracer distribution can be studied. A cold nodule is an area in the gland that does not take up the iodine. A cold nodule indicates the presence of a cyst or a potential malignant nodule. A hot nodule is a focal area of intense tracer activity indicating a hyperfunctioning thyroid nodule.

Ultrasound is the imaging procedure of choice for studying the cross-sectional anatomy of the gland. Because the thyroid is a superficial structure, ultrasound is perfect for this purpose. The thyroid size and volume can be calculated and nodules can be classified as solid or cystic. Ultrasound is also used to guide biopsy.

The two most common ways to image the parathyroid glands are nuclear imaging and ultrasound.

Nuclear imaging of the parathyroid glands can be completed in several ways. A subtraction technique involves administering technetium-99m pertechnetate, followed by thallium-201. The Tc-99m pertechnetate is taken up by the thyroid and parathyroid glands. Thallium-201 is taken up exclusively by the thyroid gland. Thyroid tissue can then be subtracted from the image, leaving only the parathyroid tissue. Alternatively, Tc-99m sestamibi can be used to detect parathyroid adenoma or hyperplasia.

Ultrasound of the parathyroid glands is often difficult because of the glands' small size, variability in location, and close proximity to the thyroid gland. As the spatial resolution of ultrasound has improved over the years, so has its utility in evaluating the parathyroid glands.

CHAPTER ELEVEN　　　NEUROIMAGING

11.0 Goals: Understanding when to order CT and MRI; identifying common CNS pathology

Objective questions:

11.1　What imaging modalities are most helpful in imaging the CNS?
11.2　When should I order a head CT?
11.3　What are the steps in examining a head CT?
11.4　When is MRI better than CT in CNS imaging?
11.5　What are the CT and MRI findings in ischemic infarction of the brain?
11.6　How can I differentiate ischemic infarction from brain tumor?
11.7　What are the findings in subdural hematoma?
11.8　What are the findings in epidural hematoma?
11.9　What are CT findings of intraparenchymal hemorrhage?
11.10　What are the findings in subarachnoid hemorrhage?
11.11　How do I evaluate the cervical spine in trauma?

11.1 What imaging modalities are most helpful in imaging the CNS?

CT and MRI are the mainstays of neuroimaging. CT is best for finding intracranial hemorrhage, middle ear/temporal bone pathology, bone lesions, and fractures of the spine or skull. CT is limited to a degree in the posterior fossa of the brain due to bone artifact. MRI is excellent for all soft tissue imaging, including the brain, spinal cord, and disks. When information is desired about vascular structures, computed tomography angiography (CTA) and magnetic resonance angiography (MRA) are excellent noninvasive ways to study the intracerebral and extracranial blood vessels. MRA is performed more often than CTA because no radiation is required. For even more detail, direct angiography of the brain is performed by a radiologist or endovascular neurosurgeon.

11.2 When should I order a head CT?

Cranial CT remains an often utilized modality in the emergency room. Its benefits include availability, quick results, and accuracy in detecting intracranial hemorrhage, including subdural, epidural, intraparenchymal, and subarachnoid bleeding. CT should never replace a thorough history and physical examination. Always consider the risk of radiation when requesting a CT. Viewing the scan on bone window settings allows for the easier detection of skull and facial bone fractures. Foreign bodies are usually obvious on CT. There is no question that MRI is more sensitive in many areas. Ischemic infarction, the most common kind of stroke, may not show up on a CT for up to 72 hours. It may be seen on CT as subtle decreased attenuation or cortical effacement as early as 5 hours after the onset of the ischemic event. According to the American Heart Association, MRI can detect ischemia within minutes of the stroke onset. Brain tumors and infections are best imaged with MRI. The pituitary gland, cranial nerves, and white matter also are best studied with magnetic resonance.

Neuroimaging

11.3 What are the steps in examining a head CT?

Steps in examining a head CT:

1. Check the name, date, and right-left orientation on the film.
2. Get a global impression of the scan; note any initial impressions, such as asymmetrical areas in the brain, blood, calcifications, or low-density areas.
3. Start a pattern search beginning with the fourth, third, and lateral ventricles and noting size, position, and symmetry.
4. At the top of the scan, compare the cortical sulci (grooves in the gray matter) from one side to the other until you have reached the skull base.
5. Look specifically for subdural or epidural hematoma.
6. Inspect the white matter tracts, including the parietal regions, the paraventricular areas, and the internal capsules.
7. Examine midline structures, beginning with the brain stem, pons, sella turcica, septum pellucidum, and corpus callosum.
8. Specifically identify the thalamus, caudate nucleus, putamen, and globus pallidus.
9. Check the paranasal sinuses for blood, fluid, or mucosal disease, and then compare the orbits.
10. Review the scalp and the skull, noting soft tissue swelling, fracture, or lytic/blastic pathology.

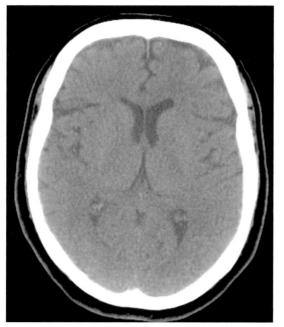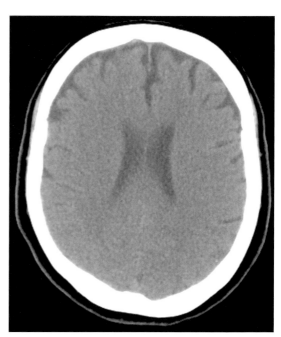

Normal head CT

Neuroimaging

11.4 When is MRI better than CT in CNS imaging?

Because MRI is expensive and not quite as readily available as CT in some medical settings, it is most often performed in the outpatient setting. This is not to say that you should not order an MRI in the emergency room or for a hospitalized patient. Ischemic infarction is detected much earlier on MRI than on CT (minutes versus hours). Ninety percent of ischemic injuries will be visible on MRI within the first 24 hours. The benefit of confirming ischemia and excluding hemorrhage early is that medical therapy can prevent ongoing tissue injury and cell death. MRI is excellent for defining the nature and extent of primary and metastatic brain tumors, cranial nerve abnormalities, pituitary adenoma, white matter diseases such as multiple sclerosis, infections, and vascular malformations such as AVM and aneurysm, and for defining congenital brain abnormalities.

Consult the radiologist if you are unsure which test to order. MRI has the benefits of no radiation, excellent anatomic detail, vascular imaging, and multiplanar capability (axial, coronal, sagittal, or any other plane can be used).

11.5 What are the CT and MRI findings in ischemic infarction of the brain?

CT findings in ischemia include loss of gray/white matter differentiation, asymmetrical effacement of the cortical sulci (mass effect), and diminished density extending from white matter to gray matter (edema). Focal round or oval hypodensity often represents lacunar infarction, which most commonly occurs in the basal ganglia, pons, or cerebellum where small penetrating blood vessels are occluded (associated with hypertension and/or diabetes). Lacunar infarction is round to oval in shape and measures up to 1.5 cm. Any area of increased density indicates hemorrhage or calcification.

MRI findings of ischemia occur because of the presence of edema. This abnormal fluid behaves differently in a magnetic field than normal brain parenchyma. On T1-weighted images, fluid will be of low signal. On inversion recovery, diffusion imaging and T2-weighted sequences, the edema fluid is high in signal. (Remember, low signal is dark gray or black on an MRI image while high signal is white.) Because of increased pressure from the edema, there will often be effacement of adjacent cortical sulci. The edema pattern will be in a wedge-shaped configuration. MRI is much more sensitive than CT in the detection of early infarction. Gradient echo MRI is also more sensitive than CT in the detection of small hemorrhages associated with infarction. Perfusion MRI demonstrates the extent of diminished parenchymal blood flow. Diffusion MRI helps in determining the age of an ischemic infarction and has greater than 90% sensitivity and specificity. Abnormal increased signal in diffusion MRI peaks at about three to five days after the infarction.

Neuroimaging

CT versus MRI in ischemic infarction of the brain (stroke)

	CT	*MRI*
Hyperacute phase (0 to 3 hours)	Normal or subtle loss of gray/white matter differentiation	Increased signal T2 Gyral swelling Sulcal effacement
Acute phase (3 to 24 hours)	Normal or subtle mass effect	Increased T2 Decreased T1
Subacute phase (1 to 7 days)	Hypodensity gray and white matter	Contrast enhancement Increased signal (diffusion)
Subacute to chronic phase (1 to 8 weeks)	Hypodensity with contrast enhancement	Gyral and white matter enhancement
Chronic phase (weeks to years)	Hypodensity matches CSF	Decreased T1/increased T2 matches CSF

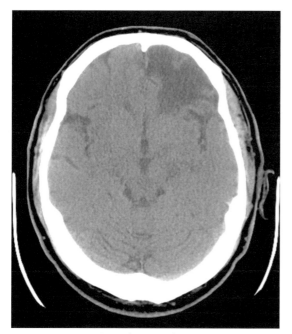

CT: Ischemic infarction

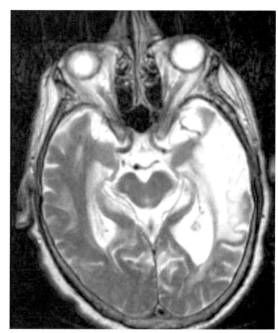

MRI: ischemic infarction

Neuroimaging

11.6 How can I differentiate ischemic infarction from brain tumor?

Ischemic infarction results from anoxia caused by arterial occlusion, most often from thrombosis and embolism. In infarction, all brain tissue supplied by the occluded artery dies in a wedge-shaped pattern, in which the apex of the wedge is the point of arterial occlusion. Therefore, white matter and gray matter are almost always affected. The wedge-shaped area appears as low density on CT secondary to edema. On MRI, edema is hypointense on T1 and hyperintense on T2. Brain tumors, whether primary or metastatic, produce edema that is often confined to the white matter.

Remember that white matter edema can occur in a wide variety of pathologies, including multiple sclerosis, vasculitis, lupus, viral encephalitis, Lyme disease, and metabolic and toxic conditions. Although tumors often enhance with contrast (iodinated contrast with CT and gadolinium with MRI), the hallmark of subacute ischemic infarction on CT is gyral enhancement. Because mass effect can occur in ischemic infarction and tumor, follow-up imaging is important. Mass effect will decrease over time with infarction and persist when there is tumor.

Summary of findings: infarction versus tumor in the brain:

Infarction:	Wedge-shaped
	White and gray matter edema
	Small amount of mass effect that resolves after 7–10 days
Brain tumor:	Round, oval, or spiculated (jagged edges)
	Edema confined to white matter
	Mass effect that persists over time

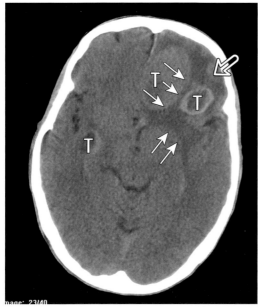 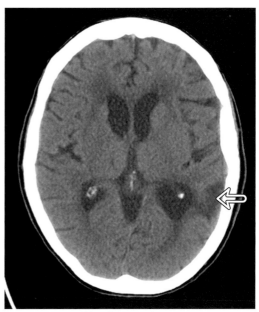

T = tumor, arrows = white matter edema,
block arrow = gray matter

Old ischemic infarction

Neuroimaging

11.7 What are the findings in subdural hematoma?

The subdural hematoma (SDH) is a favorite image shown on board examinations. The dura mater is the thickest member of the three meninges covering the brain and spinal cord. The dura adheres tightly to the inner table of the skull, but the subdural space is compliant. When blood enters this space, usually as a result of injury to the bridging veins, there is little resistance to the accumulation and spread of the hemorrhage. The blood accumulates between the dura and the arachnoid meninges. The resulting shape of the SDH is crescent: convex along the curvature of the skull and concave along the curvature of the brain.

With computed tomography, the density (whiteness, grayness, or blackness) depends upon the age of the SDH. An acute subdural hematoma (less than three days) will be white on CT. A subacute subdural (three to seven days to two to three weeks) will be gray, often matching the density of the adjacent brain (isodense SDH). A chronic subdural, blood older than two to three weeks, will be hypodense to brain, eventually matching the density of cerebrospinal fluid (black on CT).

With MRI, the crescent-shaped SDH has variable signal on T1 and T2, also dependent on the age of the blood (see table 11.8). In an acute SDH, the blood is of intermediate signal on T1 and high signal on T2. With late acute and early subacute hemorrhage there is low T2 signal. It is in this time period that I find intracranial bleeding more difficult to detect on MRI than on CT. With subacute bleeding, the SDH is of high signal on T1 and on T2. As the subdural reaches the chronic stage, the hematoma matches cerebrospinal fluid: low on T1 and high on T2. Remember that low signal is dark gray or black on the image and high signal is light gray or white.

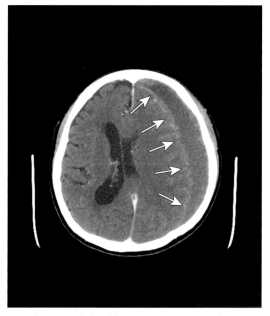

Subacute subdural hematoma (crescent shape)

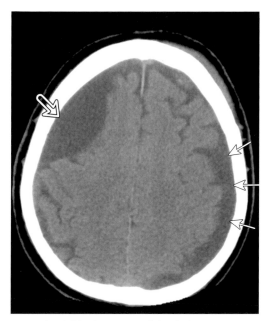

Epidural (block arrow); subdural (thin arrows)

Neuroimaging

11.8 What are the findings in epidural hematoma?

Epidural hematoma (EDH) is often included in board examinations to be recognized and distinguished from subdural bleeding. The dura adheres tightly to the inner table of the skull, so that separating the dura from the skull takes pressure. Most epidural hematomas are caused by arterial bleeding, and most result from injury to the middle meningeal artery secondary to skull fracture. As blood forces its way between the dura and the skull, a lenticular (lens-shaped), biconvex hemorrhage occurs. The hematoma is convex along the skull and is also convex toward the brain.

With CT, blood undergoes a characteristic density change as it ages. In acute EDH, the hemorrhage is dense (white). Hyperacute EDH is a situation in which there is active bleeding. In this case, active bleeding (hypodense—black) is seen mixed with the acute hemorrhage (dense—white). As blood ages, a subacute EDH (three to seven days to two to three weeks) becomes gray and isodense with the adjacent brain parenchyma. Chronic epidural hematoma is characterized by a lens-shaped low-density fluid accumulation of similar density to cerebrospinal fluid.

MRI also reflects these stages of blood degradation from intact red blood cells to the end result of hemosiderin. With MRI, six stages of hemorrhage can be recognized:

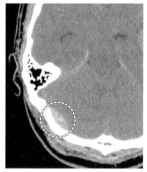

CT: acute epidural hematoma

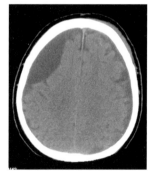

CT: chronic epidural hematoma

MRI signal in hemorrhage

Stage of hemorrhage	T1	T2
Oxyhemoglobin	Isointense	Hyperintense
Deoxyhemoglobin	Hypointense	Hypointense
Intracellular methemaglobin	Hyperintense	Hypointense
Extracellular methemaglobin	Hyperintense	Hyperintense
Seroma	Hypointense	Hyperintense
Hemosiderin	Hypointense	Hypointense

Neuroimaging

11.9 What are CT findings of intraparenchymal hemorrhage?

CT is often the first imaging procedure ordered to exclude intracranial hemorrhage. Bleeding that occurs within the brain parenchyma is often the result of trauma, hemorrhagic stroke, or rupture of a vascular malformation, such as berry aneurysm or arteriovenous malformation. Hemorrhage can also be seen in primary or metastatic brain cancer. Acute bleeding into the brain is manifested by focal increased CT density surrounded by a variable zone of low-density edema. Intracranial hemorrhage is variable in shape. It may be round or oval with relatively smooth margins, or the density may present with an irregular shape.

Hemorrhagic stroke is associated with anticoagulation therapy and hypertension. Bleeding under these circumstances most frequently occurs in the cerebellum and basal ganglia. Posttraumatic intraparenchymal hemorrhage may occur adjacent to the skull closest to the site of injury or opposite the site of injury. Bleeding on the side opposite the trauma is referred to as *contra coup hemorrhage.* Vascular malformations commonly result in subarachnoid hemorrhage in addition to intraparenchymal bleeding. An underlying tumor should be considered if a cause for the hemorrhage cannot be explained by any other mechanism, particularly if the surrounding zone of edema seems larger or out of proportion to the amount of bleeding present.

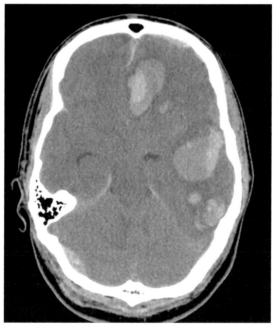

Intraparenchymal hemorrhage

Neuroimaging

11.10 What are the findings in subarachnoid hemorrhage?

Bleeding into the subarachnoid space can result in subtle findings on CT. Examining the ventricles, cisterns, and cortical sulci is the secret to recognizing subarachnoid hemorrhage (SAH). On CT, acute hemorrhage into the subarachnoid space produces hyperdensity within the normally low-density cerebrospinal fluid spaces. The hemorrhage often favors a specific CSF space, depending upon the origin of the bleeding. For example, a ruptured anterior communicating artery aneurysm most often results in high-density blood in the supra-sellar cistern. If the aneurysm is at the bifurcation of the left middle cerebral artery, the hyperdense blood will accumulate in the left sylvian cistern. Any cistern, ventricle, or cortical sulcation can become opacified with blood. Carefully examining each of these spaces and comparing the opposite side for symmetry will allow you to identify SAH.

11.11 How do I evaluate the cervical spine in trauma?

There are three basic projections obtained in a traumatic C-spine series: lateral, AP, and open-mouth odontoid views. It is important that the entire cervical spine be included on the lateral projection, from the cranio-cervical junction to the T1 vertebral body. Remember that fractures may still be present in a normal-appearing cervical spine X-ray.

Steps in evaluating the lateral cervical spine X-ray:

- ✔ Count seven cervical segments
- ✔ Check alignment (three smooth arcs)
- ✔ Measure soft tissues from the anterior spine to the airway
    Normal = 6 mm at C2 and 22 mm at C6 (6 at 2 and 22 at 6)
- ✔ Compare vertebral body heights
- ✔ Compare intervertebral disk spaces
- ✔ Assess cortex margins of each vertebra
- ✔ Assess all spinous processes
- ✔ Odontoid process (3 mm or less between C1 and odontoid)

Steps in evaluating the AP view:

- ✔ Check alignment of the spinous processes
- ✔ Evaluate for equal inter-spinous distance
- ✔ Reassess vertebral body heights

Steps in evaluating the open-mouth odontoid view:

- ✔ Make sure lateral edges of C1 and C2 aligned
- ✔ Check whether odontoid process intact
- ✔ Check for equal distance between the odontoid and lateral masses C1

CHAPTER TWELVE   IMPROVING PROFICIENCY

12.0 Goals: Gaining confidence with image interpretation and tips for board preparation

Objective questions:

12.1 I have no experience with image interpretation. Where do I begin?
12.2 I have a basic understanding of imaging, but how can I improve at recognizing pathology?
12.3 Are there additional recommended resources for learning the basics of radiology?
12.4 How should I prepare for imaging questions on board examinations?

12.1 I have no experience with image interpretation. Where do I begin?

I believe that it is easier to understand and remember reproducible processes than memorize vast quantities of facts. To understand a process like image interpretation, you must first learn how images are created. Nearly every textbook on the subject of radiology begins with a review of how the imaging modality works.

I find that to teach is to learn twice, that is, I learn best if I can read about a subject, simplify or rephrase it into my own words, and explain it to someone else. To get the best foundation for interpreting X-rays and other medical imaging studies, first learn the basics of how each modality works and then explain it to your peers.

After that, you should learn the appearance of normal anatomic structures. The best way to do this is by physically labeling the structures. (During my first several years of practice as a radiologist, attending physicians knew that I was the one interpreting their patients' films if they found normal anatomy labeled with a wax pencil.) I have found several Web sites that provide unlabeled and labeled imaging anatomy. If you can identify normal, then pathology becomes easier to recognize.

Finally, practice the art of interpretation by online quizzes. There are many excellent radiology teaching Web sites (please see section 12.3). The American College of Radiology (http://www.acr.org) has an outstanding educational series. Although it is geared toward residents, is not beyond the grasp of students who have gained some experience. Image interpretation is a skill that responds well to continuous practice but gathers rust if left alone. It is not necessary to spend hours practicing; if you attempt two or three imaging quizzes each week, your skills will grow steadily, and so will your perception abilities and confidence.

Improving Proficiency

12.2 I have a basic understanding of imaging, but how can I improve at recognizing pathology?

If you practice a reproducible pattern of analysis, you will begin to quickly recognize normal anatomy. With every imaging study, you should have a plan. In the chest, I recommend the mnemonic "MDPLOTS" (see chapter 5). In the abdomen, I suggest using the five basic radiographic densities (see chapter 6). For plain films of bones and joints, start with soft tissues, looking for swelling, foreign bodies, air, and fat displacement, then trace the cortex of each bone and finally examine the medullary cavities. Please refer to the individual chapters of this book.

As you move through your reproducible pattern search, pay close attention to *symmetry*. With obvious exceptions, such as the heart and abdominal viscera, the right and left sides of the body are mirror images of each other. Comparing them is an extremely important component of image analysis. Pathologic conditions tend to produce areas of tissue asymmetry. A very good example of symmetry analysis is in the examination of the cortical sulcations of the brain. Subtle edema or swelling will often result in flattening of the sulci on one side of the brain when compared to the other.

Size analysis is a key component of imaging interpretation. Usually you can easily recognize that a structure is larger or smaller than normal. When in doubt, measure. The cardiac diameter can be assessed by the cardio-thoracic ratio, the kidneys should be approximately the size of two and a half vertebral segments, and the liver should extend no lower than approximately two finger breadths below the costal margin (the exception is Riedel's lobe in females). Fast-growing pathology (tumor cells) results in enlargement of the affected organ. Infarction (cell death) results in scarring and therefore causes organs to shrink in size.

Shape is something that we often notice but may not give due consideration. We can generally count on normal structures to have a reliable, reproducible contour. The ventricles of the brain, the aortic arch, the superior mediastinum, the reniform shape of the kidneys and lymph nodes, and even the round shape of simple cysts are constant unless there is a pathologic process involved. In general, a round, smooth structure favors benign disease (exception metastasis), while irregular and especially spiculated margins suggest the haphazard growth of malignancy. As you learn imaging anatomy, consider and commit to memory the normal shapes and contours of body structures.

The *position* of normal structures should be assessed on every image. This fundamental idea is true in any area of the body. A good example is found in the analysis of chest X-rays. Shift of the trachea can result from a mediastinal mass (the trachea is pushed) or from volume loss caused by an obstructing mass (the trachea is pulled). The mediastinum, the heart, or the diaphragms can be pushed or pulled, depending upon whether the pathology is space-occupying or space-constricting.

Tissue density is the final, highly important factor in the perception/analysis of imaging pathology. Again, as a general rule, pathologic conditions result in an increase or a decrease in tissue density. Examples on an X-ray are high-density pathologies such as gallstones, kidney stones, calcified granulomas, arteriosclerosis, degenerative joint disease, and osteoblastic metastatic disease. On the other hand, abnormally decreased density is seen in a wide variety of pathology, such as osteoporosis, osteolytic metastatic disease, and cystic lesions that occur commonly in solid organs. Remember that the term *density* is applied to imaging studies using X-rays, *signal* is used in MRI, *intensity* is used in nuclear imaging, and *echogenicity* is used in ultrasound.

Improving Proficiency

The basics of image analysis:

- ✔ Start with a plan, a reproducible pattern of study.
- ✔ Search for areas of asymmetry.
- ✔ For all structures, whether normal anatomy or pathology, consider

> Size
> Shape
> Position
> Density/signal/intensity/echogenicity

Summary: Steps in evaluating an imaging study:

Maintain a darkened environment to optimize the ratio of light coming from the viewbox or computer screen to the background.

Review any available clinical data, history, physical findings, or lab results.

Get a first impression the instant you lay eyes on the image.

Check the image for quality. Is the image overpenetrated or underpenetrated? Are there artifacts? Is the patient rotated?

Start a pattern of search.

For joints and extremities, look for soft tissue swelling or joint effusion first.

For the chest, follow the MDPLOTS mnemonic.

In the abdomen, guide your search by the five basic radiographic densities: air, fat, soft tissue, mineral, and metal.

For all other studies, including CT, ultrasound, and MRI, identify normal anatomy. Anything left over is the pathology! I think that when you are first learning to interpret cross-sectional imaging it helps to label all structures with an erasable wax pencil. If the image is on a monitor, annotate the normal structures with letter abbreviations.

Make a conscious effort to review hidden areas, including the corners of the film.

Study all the views that you have. Pathology may be visible on only one of the views.

Communicate your findings accurately, clearly, and concisely.

Document your communication in writing.

12.3 Are there additional recommended resources for learning the basics of radiology?

The following are my favorite imaging Web sites; there are many more.

1. http://www.learningradiology.com
2. http://www.auntminnie.com
3. http://www.acr.org (ACR learning file online)
4. http://www.radiologyeducation.com/
5. http://rad.usuhs.mil/
6. http://www.radweb.org/
7. http://caseinpoint.acr.org/
8. http://www.blograd.blogspot.com
9. http://www.rad.uab.edu
10. http://www.theoralboard.com/
11. http://ultrasound.ucsf.edu/USCases.html
12. http://www.med.wayne.edu/diagRadiology/TF/TeachingFile.html

Note: These Web sites are always subject to change and may not remain active on a permanent basis. There are many more excellent sites that can be found through an Internet search engine. I recommend using online resources for two purposes: learning normal imaging anatomy and "case-of-the-day" practice.

There are many excellent books on the subject of radiology. See Further Reading for a few that I have found especially useful for medical students and interns. *Blueprints in Radiology* is designed to be a USMLE board review. When students are on my service, I lend them a copy of *Squire's Fundamentals of Radiology.*

Improving Proficiency

12.4 How should I prepare for imaging questions on board examinations?

Constructing a plan of attack for the medical imaging questions on COMLEX or USMLE can be difficult. In the weeks prior to the examination, it is not practical to read a three-hundred-page text or become engulfed in the myriad of imaging quizzes found online. My suggestion is to construct a list of 50 to 75 diagnoses that are common in medical practice and study them by searching for the cases online. Beyond this, a live board review class is ideal (my opinion). Most schools have organized board reviews, and if not, students can organize them with volunteer faculty. The following is a partial list of common diagnoses that I believe would be fair game for board exams.

Orbital blowout fracture (X-ray and CT)
Epiglottitis (X-ray)
Retropharyngeal abscess (X-ray and CT)
Acute sinusitis (X-ray and CT)
Thyroglossal duct cyst (CT and MRI)
Parotid tumor (CT and MRI)
Tripod facial bone fracture (X-ray and CT)
Ischemic brain infarction (CT and MRI)
Glioblastoma—brain (MRI)
Meningioma (MRI)
Pituitary adenoma (MRI)

Pneumoconiosis (X-ray)
Mesothelioma (X-ray and CT)
Pulmonary abscess (X-ray)
Reactivation tuberculosis (X-ray)
Pneumocystis pn (X-ray)
Pulmonary embolism (CTA)
Aortic dissection (CT and MRI)
Pneumoperitoneum (X-ray)
Small bowel obstruction (X-ray)
Colon obstruction (X-ray)
Pancreatitis (CT)

Multiple sclerosis (MRI)
Acoustic schwannoma (MRI)
Subarachnoid hemorrhage (CT)
Subdural hematoma (CT and MRI)
Epidural hematoma (CT and MRI)
Intracranial metastasis (CT and MRI)
Pneumococcal pneumonia (X-ray)
Bronchopneumonia (X-ray)
Emphysema (X-ray and CT)
Congestive heart failure (X-ray)
Pneumothorax (supine and upright X-ray)
Pleural effusion (X-ray)
Lung cancer (X-ray and CT)
Sarcoidosis (X-ray and CT)

Diverticulitis (CT)
Cholelithiasis (ultrasound)
Breast cancer (mammography)
Breast cyst (ultrasound)
AVN of the hip (MRI)
Scaphoid fracture (X-ray)
Hip fracture (X-ray and MRI)
Elbow fat pad (X-ray)
Shoulder dislocation (X-ray)
ACL tear (MRI)
Salter-Harris classification
C1 Jefferson fracture (X-ray)
Lisfranc fracture (X-ray)
Calcaneus fracture (X-ray and CT)

PART THREE

Imaging Anatomy and Pathology

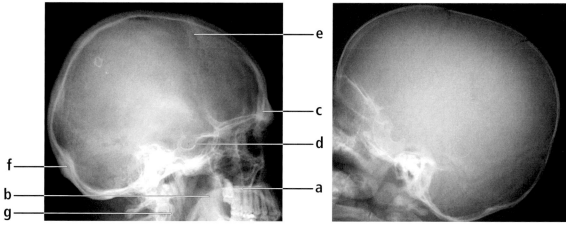

1a. Name these structures

1b. What is your diagnosis?

Answers 1a.

a. hard palate
b. soft palate
c. frontal sinus
d. sella turcica
e. coronal suture
f. external occipital protuberance
g. anterior arch of C1

Answer 1b.

Linear parietal skull fracture
(note: sharp radiolucent line without branching)

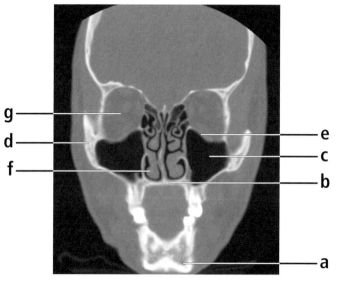

2a. Name these structures

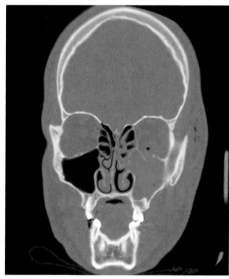

2b. What is your diagnosis?

Answers 2a

a. Mandible
b. alveolar ridge
c. maxillary sinus
d. zygoma
e. orbital floor
f. inferior turbinate
g. optic nerve

Answer 2b.

Blowout fracture left orbit
(note: air in left orbit and air in subcutaneous tissue)

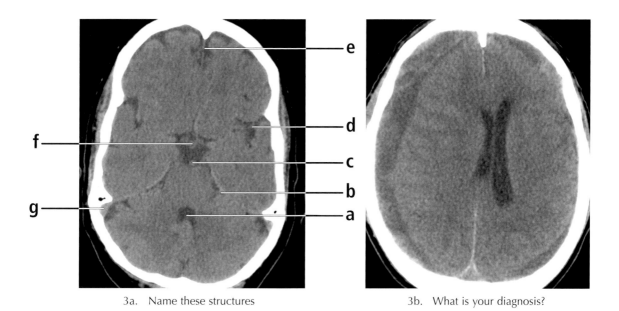

3a. Name these structures

3b. What is your diagnosis?

Answers 3a.

a. fourth ventricle
b. tentorium
c. basilar artery
d. sylvian fissure cistern
e. falx cerebri
f. optic chiasm
g. sigmoid sinus

Answer 3b.

CT bilateral subdural hematoma
(mixed chronic and subacute)

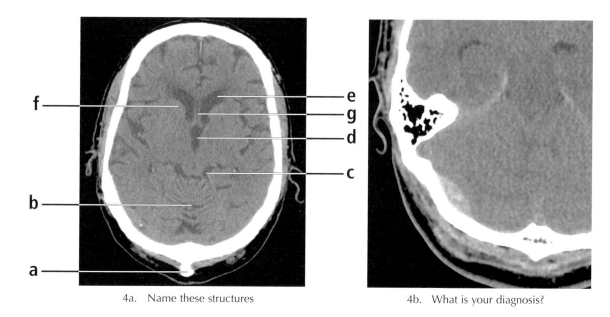

4a. Name these structures

4b. What is your diagnosis?

Answers 4a.

a. external occipital protuberance
b. vermian folia of cerebellum
c. quadrigeminal plate cistern
d. third ventricle
e. anterior horn lateral ventricle
f. head of caudate nucleus
g. septum pellucidum

Answer 4b.

Right occipital epidural hematoma
(note: lens shape of the hemorrhage)

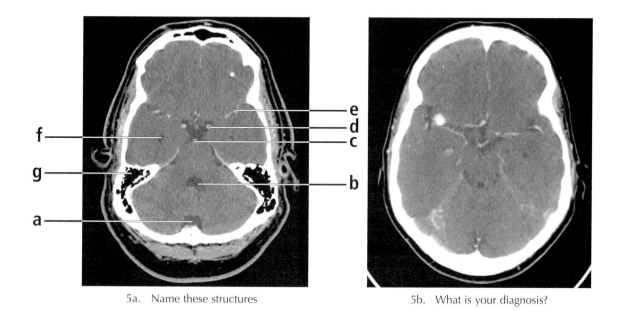

5a. Name these structures

5b. What is your diagnosis?

Answers 5a.

a. superior cerebellar cistern
b. fourth ventricle
c. basilar artery
d. internal carotid artery
e. middle cerebral artery
f. temporal horn of lateral ventricle
g. mastoid air cells

Answer 5b.

Right middle cerebral artery aneurysm

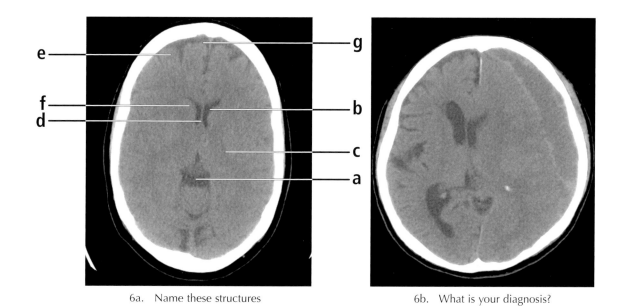

6a. Name these structures

6b. What is your diagnosis?

Answers 6a.
_____

a. superior cerebellar cistern
b. anterior horn lateral ventricle
c. posterior limb internal capsule
d. septum pellucidum
e. frontal cortex
f. head of caudate nucleus
g. posterior limb internal capsule

Answer 6b.
_____

Left subdural hematoma
(note: semilunar shape and left-to-right midline shift)

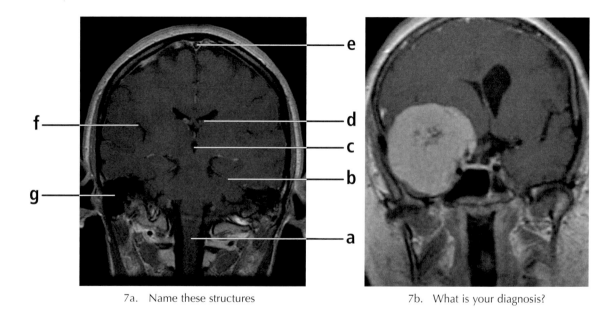

7a. Name these structures

7b. What is your diagnosis?

Answers 7a.

a. cervical spinal cord
b. tentorium
c. third ventricle
d. choroid plexus (lateral ventricle)
e. superior sagittal sinus
f. sylvian fissure
g. mastoid air cells

Answer 7b.

Large right temporal meningioma
(coronal MRI with gadolinium)

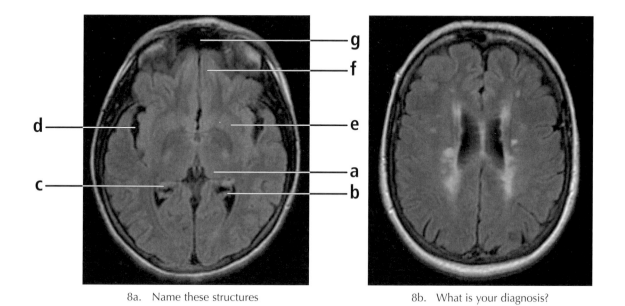

8a. Name these structures

8b. What is your diagnosis?

Answers 8a.

a. thalamus
b. trigone or atrium of lateral ventricles
c. choroids plexus
d. sylvian fissure
e. basal ganglia
f. frontal lobe
g. frontal sinus

Answer 8b.

FLAIR sequence demonstrating multiple sclerosis

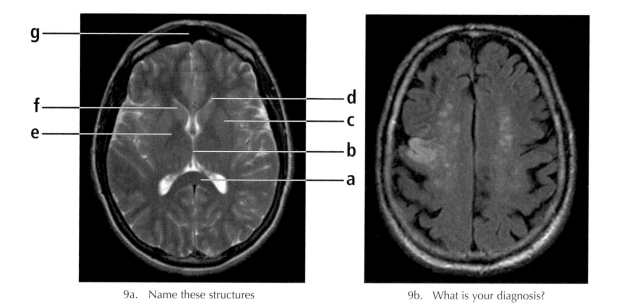

9a. Name these structures

9b. What is your diagnosis?

Answers 9a.

a. splenium of corpus callosum
b. third ventricle
c. putamen and globus pallidus
d. anterior horn lateral ventricle
e. genu of internal capsule
f. head of caudate nucleus
g. frontal sinus

Answer 9b.

Ischemic infarction right midparietal lobe
(note: degenerative white matter)

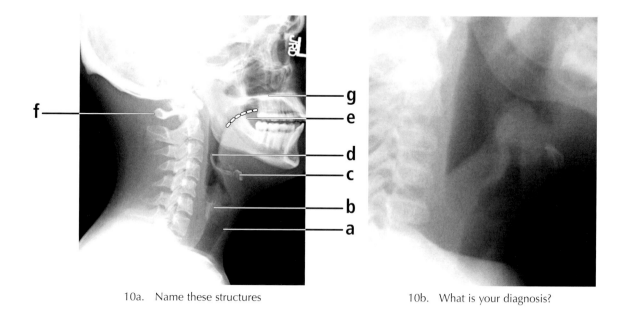

10a. Name these structures

10b. What is your diagnosis?

Answers 10a.

a. trachea
b. thyroid cartilage
c. hyoid bone
d. epiglottis
e. tongue
f. posterior arch C1
g. hard palate

Answer 10b.

Acute epiglottitis

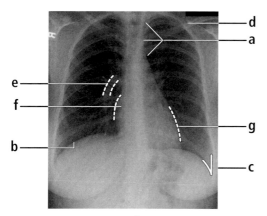

11a. Name these structures

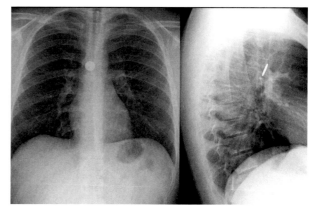

11b. What is your diagnosis?

Answers 11a.

a. mediastinum
b. right diaphragm
c. costophrenic angle
d. clavicle
e. right pulmonary artery
f. right atrium
g. left ventricle

Answer 11b.

Foreign body (coin) trachea

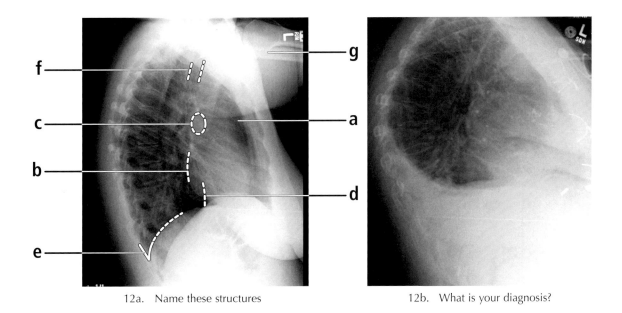

12a. Name these structures

12b. What is your diagnosis?

Answers 12a.

a. retrosternal clear space
b. inferior vena cava
c. left ventricle
d. left hemi diaphragm
e. posterior costophrenic angle
f. trachea
g. right pulmonary artery

Answer 12b.

Pleural effusion
(note: fluid with meniscus posterior costophrenic angle)

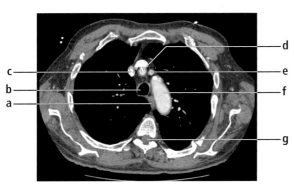

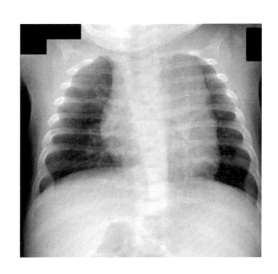

13a.   Name these structures

13b.   What is your diagnosis?

Answers 13a.

a. esophagus
b. trachea
c. superior vena cava
d. brachiocephalic artery
e. left common carotid artery
f. aortic arch
g. thoracic spinal cord

Answer 13b.

Normal thymic shadow

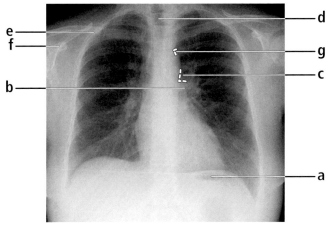

14a. Name these structures

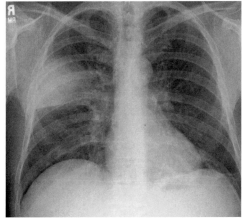

14b. What is your diagnosis?

Answers 14a.

a. stomach bubble
b. left main pulmonary artery
c. aorticopulmonary window
d. trachea
e. first rib
f. coracoid process of scapula
g. aortic arch

Answer 14b.

Right upper lobe consolidation
(most likely bacterial pneumonia)

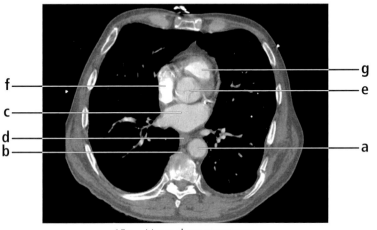

15a. Name these structures

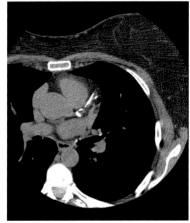

15b. What is your diagnosis?

Answers 15a.

a. descending aorta
b. azygos vein
c. left atrium
d. esophagus
e. aortic root
f. right atrium
g. right ventricle

Answer 15b.

Calcification coronary arteries

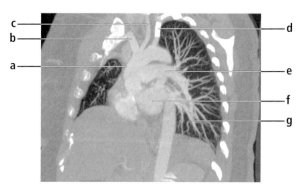

16a. Name these structures

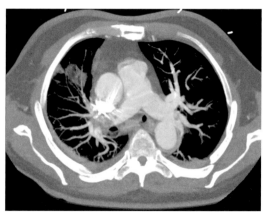

16b. What is your diagnosis?

Answers 16a.

a. ascending aortic arch
b. brachiocephalic artery
c. left common carotid artery
d. left subclavian artery with stent
e. left main pulmonary artery
f. left atrium
g. left lower lobe pulmonary veins

Answer 16b.

Pulmonary embolism, right pulmonary artery
(note: bilateral pleural effusion and right upper lobe pneumonia)

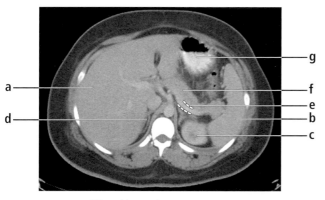

a ———

d ———

g

f

e

b

c

17a. Name these structures

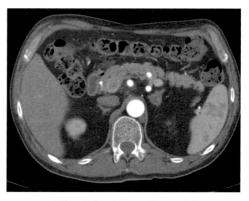

17b. What is your diagnosis?

Answers 17a.

a. right lobe of liver
b. spleen
c. left kidney
d. right adrenal gland
e. splenic vein
f. pancreas
g. stomach

Answer 17b.

Left adrenal nodule

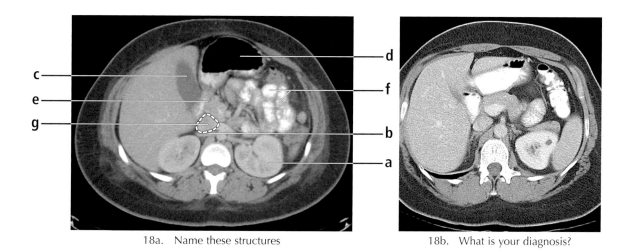

18a. Name these structures

18b. What is your diagnosis?

Answer 18a.

a. left kidney
b. right renal artery
c. gallbladder
d. stomach
e. duodenum
f. small bowel
g. inferior vena cava

Answer 18b.

Simple cyst, left kidney

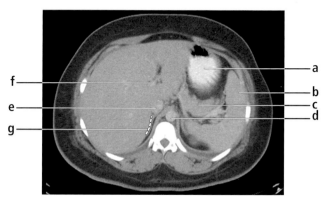

f ——
e ——
g ——

a
b
c
d

19a. Name these structures

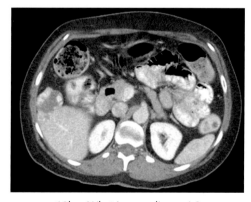

19b. What is your diagnosis?

Answers 19a.

a. stomach
b. spleen
c. tail of pancreas
d. aorta
e. inferior vena cava
f. portal vein
g. right adrenal gland

Answer 19b.

Enhancing liver metastasis

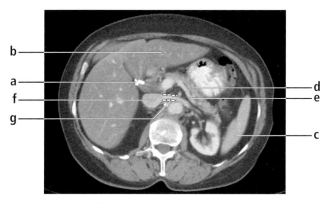

20a. Name these structures

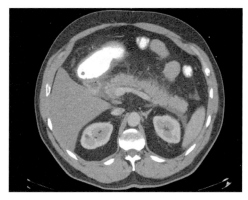

20b. What is your diagnosis?

Answers 20a.

a. surgical clips from cholecystectomy
b. left lobe of liver
   (note: diminished density related to fatty infiltration)
c. spleen
d. pancreas
e. splenic vein
f. inferior vena cava
g. left renal vein

Answer 20b.

Acute pancreatitis
(note: stranding of fat adjacent to pancreas)

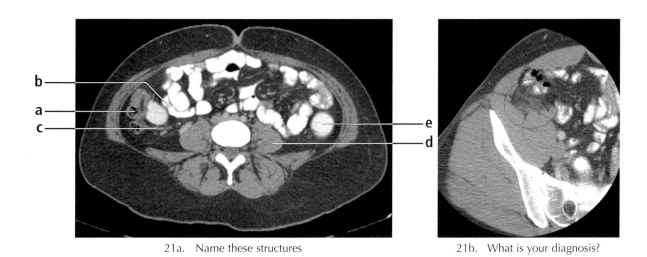

21a. Name these structures

21b. What is your diagnosis?

Answers 21a.

a. cecum
b. terminal small bowel
c. appendix
d. psoas muscle
e. descending colon

Answer 21b.

Early acute appendicitis
(note: inflammatory stranding in mesenteric fat)

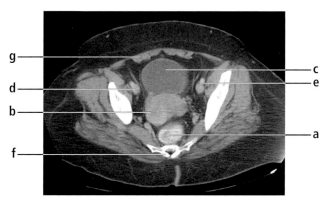

22a. Name these structures

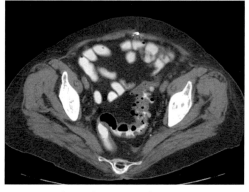

22b. What is your diagnosis?

Answers 22a.

a. rectum
b. uterus
c. urinary bladder
d. right common iliac vein
e. left common iliac artery
f. sacrum
g. rectus abdominus muscle

Answer 22b.

Sigmoid diverticulosis

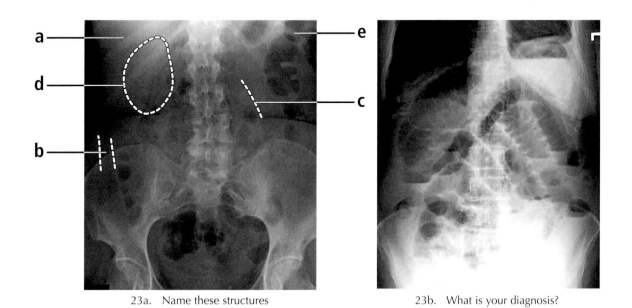

23a. Name these structures

23b. What is your diagnosis?

Answers 23a.

a. liver
b. properitoneal fat stripe
c. psoas muscle
d. right kidney
e. splenic flexure of colon

Answer 23b.

Small bowel obstruction
(note: asynchronous air-fluid levels)

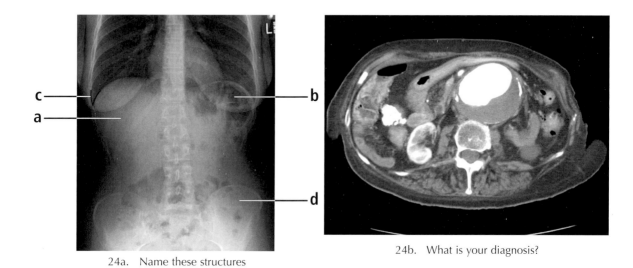

24a. Name these structures

24b. What is your diagnosis?

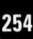

Answers 24a.

a. liver
b. splenic flexure of colon
c. right costophrenic angle
d. left iliac crest

Answer 24b.

Abdominal aortic aneurysm

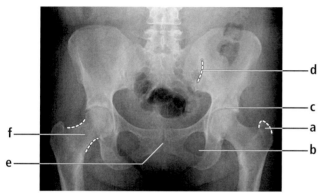

25a. Name these structures

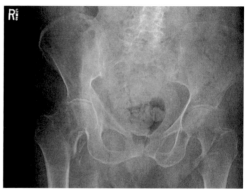

25b. What is your diagnosis?

Answers 25a.

a. great trochanter
b. obturator foramen
c. acetabulum
d. sacroiliac joint
e. symphysis pubis
f. femoral neck

Answer 25b.

Comminuted intracapsular fracture, right femoral neck

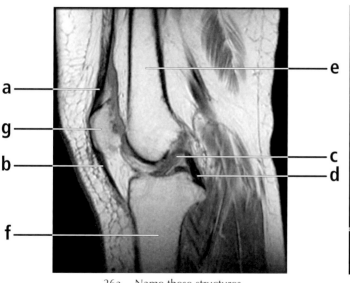

26a. Name these structures

26b. What is your diagnosis?

Answers 26a.

a. quadriceps tendon
b. patellar tendon
c. anterior cruciate ligament
d. posterior cruciate ligament
e. femur
f. tibia
g. patella

Answer 26b.

Anterior cruciate ligament disruption with large effusion

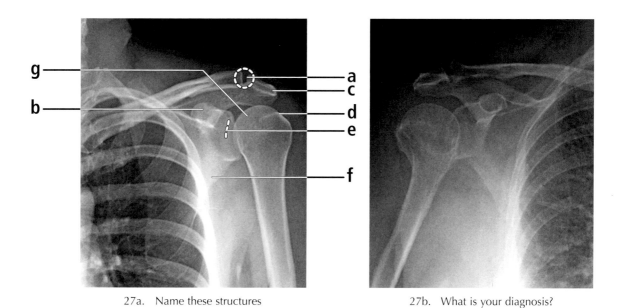

27a. Name these structures

27b. What is your diagnosis?

Answers 27a.
_____

a. acromioclavicular joint
b. coracoid process
c. acromion process
d. greater tuberocity of humerous
e. glenoid
f. scapula
g. humeral head

Answer 27b.
_____

Fracture, right humeral neck

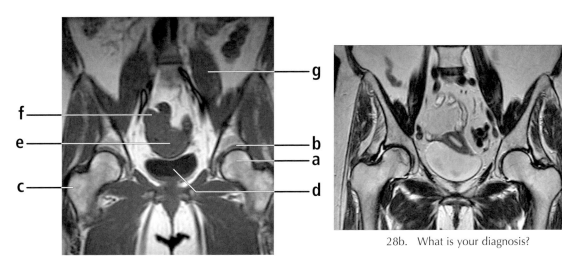

28a. Name these structures

28b. What is your diagnosis?

Answers 28a.

a. femoral head
b. acetabulum
c. greater trochanter
d. urinary bladder
e. uterus
f. right ovary
g. psoas muscle

Answer 28b.

Avascular necrosis, right femoral head

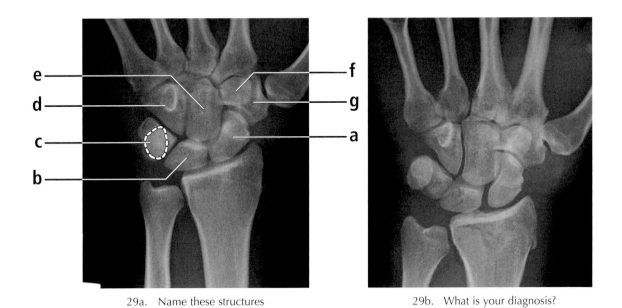

29a.   Name these structures

29b.   What is your diagnosis?

Answers 29a.

a. scaphoid
b. lunate
c. pisiform
d. hamate
e. capitate
f. trapezoid
g. trapezium

Answer 29b.

Comminuted fracture distal radial metaphysis with scapholunate dissociation

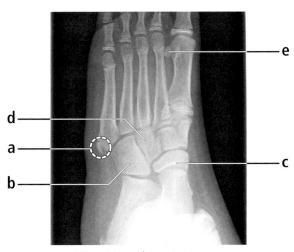

30a. Name these structures

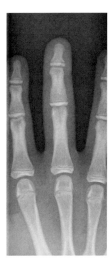

30b. What is your diagnosis?

Answers 30a.

a. growth plate proximal fifth metatarsal
b. cuboid
c. navicular
d. medial cuneiform
e. sesamoid

Answer 30b.

Salter-Harris type III fracture, distal phalanx

Further Reading

Brant, William E., and Clyde A. Helms. *Fundamentals of Diagnostic Radiology.* 2nd ed. Baltimore: Williams and Wilkins, 1999.

Davis, Ryan W., Mitchell S. Komaiko, and Barry D. Pressman. *Blueprints in Radiology.* Malden, MA: Blackwell, 2003.

Erkonen, William E., and Wilbur L. Smith. *Radiology 101: The Basics and Fundamentals of Imaging.* 2nd ed. Philadelphia: Lippincott Williams and Wilkins, 2005.

Mettler, Fred A. *Essentials of Radiology.* 2nd ed. Philadelphia: Elsevier Saunders, 2005.

Novelline, Robert A. *Squire's Fundamentals of Radiology.* 6th ed. Cambridge, MA: Harvard University Press, 2004.

Ouellette, Hugue, and Patrice Tétrault. *Clinical Radiology Made Ridiculously Simple.* 2nd ed. Miami: Medmaster, 2006.

Raby, Nigel, Laurence Berman, and Gerald De Lacey. *Accident and Emergency Radiology: A Survival Guide.* 2nd ed. Philadelphia: Elsevier Saunders, 2005.

Index

Index

86, 93; radiographic density, 24; in scrotum (hydrocele), 124; serous, in pleural effusion, 78, 82; in soft tissues, 101, 157; in subarachnoid hemorrhage, 192; transudate, 69; ultrasound for imaging, 48, 50, 112, 127, 137; water, 86

fluorodeoxyglucose (FDG), 61

fluoroscopy: with barium studies, 136; in chest, 60; in colon, 134; in upper GI, 130

foreign body: in abdomen, 108; aspiration, 68–69; in chest, 6, 68–69; in elbow, 12; in esophagus, 7, 128; in forearm, 12; in hand, 13; in head, 177; in lower leg, 15; in lungs, 69; metal, in chest, 102; in small bowel, 104; in soft tissues near bone, 147, 196; in thorax, 92; in upper abdomen, 92; in upper arm 12; in wrist, 13

fractures: acetabulum, 14, 40, 41, 44, 156, 203; abdomen, 102; angulation, 146; articular involvement, 146; bone scanning for imaging, 158; C1 Jefferson, 203; calcaneus, 16, 42, 44, 203; clavicle, 11; comminution, 146; CT for imaging, 40, 44, 156, 177; describing, 146–47; displacement, 146; elbow, 12; facial bone, 41, 156, 166, 168–73, 177, 202; foot, 15; glenoid/scapular, 11; growth plate, 148–49; healing, 143; joint, 20; Lisfranc, 203; long bone, 146; longitudinal, 146; lumbar spine, 162; MRI for imaging, 157; oblique, 146; open or closed, 146; orbital blowout, 167, 169, 170, 202; Salter-Harris classification, 148–49; scaphoid, 203; shoulder, 12; skull, 4, 177, 188; spiral, 146; sternal, 156; talar, 156; thorax, 92; tibial plateau, 15, 40, 156; transverse, 146; tripod, 172, 202; wrist, 13; X-rays for imaging, 24, 144–45

free intraperitoneal air. *See* pneumoperitoneum

fungus: as cause of cystic cavitation, 97; fungal infection, 88; fungal pneumonia, 97

gallbladder: abscess, 110; bile within, 48; disease, 112; HIDA scan for imaging, 137; porcelain gallbladder, 32, 102; ultrasound for imaging, 50, 110, 127, 137. *See also* gallstones

gallstones, 102; ultrasound for imaging, 48, 112; X-rays for imaging, 197

gastric obstruction, 130

gastroesophageal reflux disease (GERD), 128

gastrointestinal (GI) tract, 125–41; barium enema, 126, 134, 136, 140–41; barium esophagram, 126, 128–29, 136, 139; cancer, 126, 136; colitis, ulcerative, 140–41; colon, 134, 140; colonoscopy, 134; CT, 126; diverticulitis, 9, 10, 19, 106, 110, 126, 130, 203; diverticulum (*see* diverticulum); endoscopy, 134, 136; esophageal cancer, 7, 62, 128, 139; fluoroscopy, 60, 134; gallbladder, 137; gastric obstruction, 130; gastroesophageal reflux disease (GERD), 128; liver, 137; pancreas, 137; polyps, 141; reflux, 7; small intestine, 104–5, 132–33, 136; spleen, 137; ulcer, 139; upper GI, 126, 130, 136, 139; X-rays for imaging, 126

Index

volvulus, 106; sigmoid, 106